Alzheimer's Disease

Prevention Strategies & Ways to Slow Progression

Lisa Byrd
PhD, FNP-BC, GNP-BC,
Gerontologist

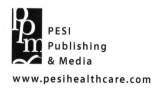

PESI
Publishing
& Media

www.pesihealthcare.com

Copyright © 2014 Lisa Byrd
Published by
PESI Publishing & Media
PESI, Inc.
3839 White Avenue
Eau Claire, WI 54703

Printed in the United States of America

Cover Design: Matt Pabich
Editing: Blair Davis
Layout: Yvonne Kuter

ISBN: 9781937661397

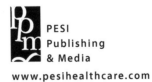

PESI
Publishing
& Media
www.pesihealthcare.com

PREFACE

We all want to live a long and healthy life — enjoying good physical health, as well as mental health, into our old age. But there are certain diseases that older individuals are more predisposed to acquiring, Alzheimer's disease (AD) being one. AD is a progressive, neurodegenerative disorder that attacks the brain, causes problems with remembering, results in memory loss, affects thinking and language skills, and eventually leads to behavioral and physical changes and even death. Thus, it is not surprising that people would like to find ways to prevent this devastating disease and/or slow the progression in those individuals who have it. While many "prevention" strategies are questionable, some have shown promise. This book presents several strategies that have been proposed to help prevent as well as slow the progression of the cognitive decline and behavioral issues that are common in individuals with AD.

First, let's examine how prevalent the problem is. According to reports in 2011, AD affects more than 5 million people in the United States. Approximately 200,000 people under the age of 65 years have the early-onset form of the disease. A larger number of individuals have decreased cognitive function, which is often referred to as mild cognitive impairment (MCI), and frequently evolves into full-blown dementia. It is projected that by 2050, AD may affect 11 to 16 million persons in the United States (Anderson, 2014).

Researchers are looking for a cure, but a significant amount of research is also being done on ways to slow the disease as well as prevent it. This book discusses the basic concepts of AD and present strategies to prevent and slow its progression, based on research, practice, and the author's professional experience.

Sections of this book were adapted from my previous book, *Caregiver Survival 101: Strategies to Manage Problematic Behaviors Presented in Individuals with Dementia*, also published by PESI, Inc.

TABLE OF CONTENTS

Alzheimer's disease affects a significant number of older individuals, and because the disorder is being diagnosed more accurately, the population size is expected to continue to increase. This chapter presents a discussion of the impact of AD on the population in the United States and the current cost of care.

Mild cognitive impairment (MCI) can be the beginning of AD, as well as other forms of dementia in an older person. This chapter discusses the pathophysiology of MCI and how the symptoms present in an elder.

This chapter discusses the pathophysiology of AD, risk factors for developing the disorder, presenting symptoms, how to diagnose AD, and current treatments.

Early-onset AD affects younger adults — sometimes those as young as 40 years. This form of AD usually has a faster progression than late-onset AD (which typically occurs after the age of 65) and often runs in families. This chapter presents a discussion of early-onset AD and how it affects the individual and family.

Researchers are proposing that there are many healthy ways to prevent MCI, AD, and vascular dementia. This chapter discusses current research suggesting healthy-brain lifestyle and exercise strategies.

This chapter discusses techniques to prevent AD, including brain-healthy dietary plans and the top 10 brain super-foods, exercise, and other lifestyle strategies.

Chapter 7: Slowing Alzheimer's Disease **121**

Alzheimer's disease is a progressive disorder, but individuals may be able to slow the progression through various techniques. This chapter presents strategies to help slow the cognitive decline and diminish or prevent behavioral issues.

Chapter 8: Family Matters **153**

When a person develops AD, many changes occur within the family. The person with the disease and the family as a whole must develop an understanding of what is occurring and create strategies to manage these changes. Conflict can occur when family members do not wish to accept the facts about the likely progression of decline. This chapter presents a discussion of common family issues and offers suggestions for their management.

Chapter 9: Taking Care of Business **167**

This chapter elaborates on ways to manage legal and financial affairs, as well as how a person may plan for his or her health care through advance directives.

References 185

About the Author 193

INTRODUCTION

Imagine waking up to start your day and remembering all the things you have to do during a busy day, beginning with getting the kids ready for school, but the kids aren't in bed — you can't even find the beds or the kids. It seems strange that your room is not the way you remembered it being when you went to sleep the night before. There are many people around, and they tell you that breakfast is in 20 minutes and you need to get ready and come to the dining room. Would you feel confused, agitated, and possibly angry? This is the situation for many individuals with AD whose memories are from their distant past. They may not remember that they now reside in a nursing home or that their kids have grown up and moved away.

Individuals who have AD have a physical disease, but the symptoms are expressed cognitively and psychologically, with memory impairments, issues understanding things, and possibly changes in personality. Having to depend on others to provide the most basic needs can make a person insecure, suspicious, paranoid, and possibly cause him or her to act differently, even aggressively. An individual's life may become an open book to the people who assist with care: caregivers know how the person slept, who visited, what the person keeps in the closet, and even if he or she has had a bowel movement. AD causes an individual to have limited ability to protect him- or herself. It's quite a vulnerable place to be, isn't it?

This vulnerability means that a person may need to make a special effort to ensure that he or she is protected and feels safe — not just physically safe, but emotionally safe as well. When dealing with someone who has AD, accept the person without judgment. Show respect and dignity. Allow

1

the individual to express his or her feelings openly. Listen and offer support. Be patient. Help him or her to feel that there is nothing to fear.

It is important to remember that every individual will react to situations in different ways. Some caregivers and relatives of individuals with AD will try to be controlling, some will be indecisive and unable to make decisions, and some may not be helpful and alienate others. Often, the problem is lack of understanding and an inability to cope with the change. However, some families find that having a family member with AD may bring a new kind of closeness as they work together to deal with stressful situations. Some people may even show strengths that they never knew they had (Alzheimer Society of Canada, 2012). This book explains what AD is, its impact, ways to cope and manage, and ways to lessen the effects and possibly slow or prevent the disease.

Chapter 1

IMPACT ON SOCIETY OF ALZHEIMER'S DISEASE

Alzheimer's disease affects a significant number of older individuals, and because the disorder is being diagnosed more accurately, the population size is expected to continue to increase. This chapter presents a discussion of the impact of AD on the population in the United States and the current cost of care.

Mom was a special person — she raised two daughters on her own. She worked the night shift and made many sacrifices so we could go to a private school and have the things we needed and wanted. We lost her after 10 years of her illness. It was devastating to see her change from a strong, vital woman who everyone depended upon into someone who no longer remembered I was her daughter. Sometimes I became her friend, sometimes I was her nurse, and other times I was the daughter she knew. It is devastating to see her decline, to see her become dependent upon others for even the simplest daily tasks. A true understanding of the disease can truly be known when you have "walked the walk." Living with a disease you have little control over and losing the parent you once knew can be devastating. As someone who has walked the walk and worn those shoes, the best plan of action is to learn all you can about the problem, attempt to discover ways to slow or prevent the problem, and learn ways to manage the problem.

Alzheimer disease is an acquired disorder affecting a person's cognition and behavior. An individual's ability to think, remember, and reason become impaired and, eventually, the progression of the disease affects the person's ability to care for him- or herself and to be independent (Anderson, 2014). AD is physiological disease, an irreversible, progressive brain disorder. In most cases, the symptoms first appear after age 60, but a small number of individuals may develop an "early-onset AD," presenting as early as in the 30s, although this is not common and represents only 4% of all people with AD (Alzheimer's Association, 2014j). Approximately 35.6 million people worldwide live with some type of dementia, AD being the most common, accounting for 60 to 70% of all dementias (World Health Organization, 2012). It is estimated that the number of people with dementia will increase to 65.7 million by 2030 and 115.4 million by 2050 (Kluger, 2010). Estimates vary, but experts suggest that in 2013, as many as 5.2 million Americans had been diagnosed with AD (Alzheimer's Association, 2014b).

A diagnosis of AD can impact a person's life markedly. One of the biggest hurdles is losing one's independence. In addition, there are expected physical and mental changes caused by the disease that can affect mood, change one's appearance, diminish positive self-image, and reduce self-esteem. This can lead to depression, anxiety, and social isolation. AD can affect one's ability to function and care for him- or herself. Initially, there may be problems with remembering recent events, inability to remember names or faces, and possibly becoming lost in familiar places. As the disease progresses, an individual may become confused and feel disoriented and unable to make sound decisions. A person with AD may be required to modify work activities and his or her environment. As the disease progresses, these issues may cause an individual to be unable to work, which may lead to a major change in lifestyle and financial difficulty.

In the early stages, individuals may be able to stay independent. They can recognize they are having issues and compensate themselves or with the assistance of a spouse of other family member or close friend. As the disease begins to progress, simple tasks may take longer to accomplish, and daily activities may become difficult to manage. If things can be done a little differently to help the individual remain independent for as long as possible, this is recommended. As AD continues to progress and impact daily life, many individuals feel a loss of control and increased anxiety about what is to come. A person with AD often experiences mood changes and feelings of anger, depression, confusion, loneliness, and frustration, especially when first diagnosed. These feelings are normal.

The best plan of action for someone with AD is to educate him- or herself about the disease, develop a plan of care to meet his or her individual needs, stay as independent as possible for as long as possible, and enjoy life. It's also important for the person with AD to take care of business by getting legal and financial affairs in order and deciding how he or she would like his or her health care directed when the person can no longer make logical decisions (an advance directive). These practical issues are discussed in Chapter 9, "Taking Care of Business."

Some of the biggest fears for families of an individual with AD are that their loved one will experience general health problems and suffer physical decline. Another major fear is that Alzheimer's will rob the family of who the person once was: The natural course of the disease alters an individual's ability to communicate and function independently and essentially changes the person the family knows and loves (Rattue, 2011).

Living with and caring for a person with AD — spending time with him or her, providing needed nurturing and love — can be rewarding. Every person who develops AD will experience declines, but the behaviors, need for care, and rate of decline will vary from one individual to another; however, there seems to be a general pattern. Caregivers should strive to maintain their relationship to the individual and are fortunate when changes in relating are minimal; caregivers should be prepared to discover ways to manage and be willing to improvise to connect with their loved ones, whether it's on an emotional level or in just meeting the person's physical needs. AD and other dementias have a significant impact on both those diagnosed and the family. As AD progresses, the individual and family may find their roles change, which may be difficult to accept. Family members may have to assume different responsibilities. A child may become the "parent" to a mother or father, and a spouse may have to take a more parental role with his or her partner — each situation is different and depends on many factors. Being the sole caregiver of a person with AD can be incredibly stressful, as well as lonely and isolating, especially if the person has reached a stage of disease that requires 24-hour care and in situations where he or she is unable to communicate properly, experiences declines in both cognition and physical functioning, or becomes aggressive and abusive.

Impact of Alzheimer's Disease

At present, some 5.4 million Americans live with a diagnosis of AD. The cost of caring for people with Alzheimer's is $200 billion, with $140 billion of it due to Medicare and Medicaid expenses. With the graying of the baby boomers, projections are that by 2050, some 16 million people will have the disease, and if nothing is done, the cost will explode to $1.1 trillion (Braunstein, 2013). The average individual with AD or any other form of dementia who has Medicare has costs that are three times higher than for those for Medicare clients without AD; the average Medicaid costs for seniors with Alzheimer's and other dementias are 19 times higher than the average per-person Medicaid spending for all other seniors (Alzheimer's Association, 2014b). These increased costs are due to the complications associated with AD, such as falls, behavioral problems necessitating medication, and other problems requiring care when the person can no longer care for him- or herself (see **Figure 1-1.**).

Figure 1-1. 2013 Cost of Care for Alzheimer's Disease in the United States (Alzheimer's Association, 2014b)

- $142 billion for Medicare & Medicaid
  - » Hospital care
  - » Nursing home care
  - » Hospice services
  - » Medications
- Out-of-pocket expenses: Insurance co-pays (including medication co-pays), homecare services, sitters, assisted living facilities, etc.
- Other: Caregivers missing work to care for the individual with AD, additional supplies necessary for care, etc.

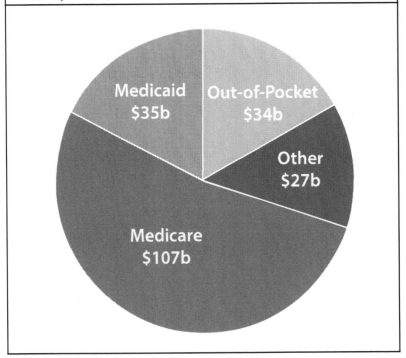

What is Alzheimer's Disease?

Alzheimer's disease is a physical disorder affecting the brain, with psychological symptoms: problems remembering, thinking, and eventually affecting one's ability to function. AD has been around for many years, and in the past had been referred to by many other names, including *senile dementia, organic brain syndrome*, and others. A better understanding of the true nature of the disease is attributed to Dr. Alois Alzheimer, who found evidence of the physiological effects on the brain in the early 1900s. Dr. Alzheimer noticed changes in the brain tissue of a female patient under his care who died of an unusual mental illness. Symptoms included memory loss, language disturbances, and unpredictable behaviors. After the woman's death, Dr. Alzheimer examined her brain and discovered many abnormal clumps (amyloid plaques) and tangled bundles of fibers (neurofibrillary tangles). The plaques and tangles within the brain are two of the main features of AD. Another physical finding in the brain of an individual with AD is a loss of connections between nerve cells (neurons). Although little is known about how the AD process begins, research suggests that damage to the brain caused by the disease may start a decade or more before problems become evident. During the period before symptoms emerge, toxic changes are taking place in the brain (National Institute on Aging, 2012; National Institutes of Health, 2013).

In the initial stages of AD, abnormal deposits of proteins (amyloid plaques) begin forming near the neurons and these proteins form tangles throughout the brain. These abnormalities within the brain affect the neurotransmitters (chemicals in the neurons that enable cells to communicate across tiny gaps called synapses [Dezell & Hill, 2013]), and this leads to an imbalance of these chemicals. Over time, neurons lose their ability to function appropriately and communicate with one other; eventually, they die, and, in combination with the chemical imbalance, this leads to changes in behavior and personality. As AD progresses, the microscopic damage spreads to a structure in the brain called the hippocampus, which is essential in forming memories. As more neurons die, more areas of the brain are involved and begin to atrophy (shrink). By the final stage of Alzheimer's, damage is widespread, and overall, the brain atrophies significantly (National Institute on Aging, 2012).

Among people older than 65 years, "late-onset" AD is the most common cause of dementia. Dementia ranges in severity from mild cognitive impairment (when a person may begin forgetting details, has trouble maintaining a conversation, becomes lost in familiar places, and/or begins developing personality changes) to the most severe stage (when he or she becomes completely dependent on others for basic activities of daily living, including mobility, bathing, dressing, eating, and toileting).

Is There Any Treatment for Alzheimer's Disease?

Currently there are four FDA-approved medications to treat AD symptoms. These medications help individuals retain more cognitive function (thinking, remembering, and speaking) by promoting maintenance of chemical balance within the brain, which helps the person stay independent and be able to carry out activities of daily living for a longer time. Medications can also help diminish some of the behavioral and personality changes associated with the disease. These medications do not stop or reverse AD, but appear to improve symptoms for a period of a few months to a few years. In the early stages, the cholinesterase inhibitor class of medications (donepezil [Aricept], rivastigmine [Exelon], and galantamine [Razadyne]) is used to maintain an appropriate level of acetylcholine. In the middle to late stages of AD, another medication is added to regulate glutamate levels — memantine (Namenda; National Institute on Aging, 2012; NINDS, 2014).

Can Alzheimer's Disease Be Prevented?

There is some epidemiologic evidence suggesting that there may be ways to reduce the risk of developing AD and slow the progression of AD in its early stages. Whereas the mainstay of management of AD includes medications to slow the progression, a healthy and active lifestyle and developing a routine will help slow the progression as well as diminish problematic behaviors. In individuals who do not show signs of the disease, a healthy lifestyle, including the following, can help reduce the risk of developing AD (Honea et al., 2009; Rolland et al., 2010):

- Physical activity
- Exercise
- Cardiorespiratory fitness
- Diet
- Mental stimulation

What Research Is Being Done?

The National Institute of Neurological Disorders and Stroke (NINDS) is su   how abnormalities in tau proteins create the characteristic neurofibrillary tangles, and the chemical imbalances caused by the plaques and tangles. Other research is exploring ways to prevent AD and slow its progression and the impact of risk factors associated with the development of AD. Researchers are also developing and testing new and novel therapies that can relieve the symptoms of AD and potentially lead to a cure (NINDS, 2014).

The Hope for Future Medications

Currently, there are five FDA-approved Alzheimer's medications that treat the symptoms of the disease, temporarily helping with memory and thinking problems. However, as stated, these medications do not prevent or treat the underlying causes of AD. New medications are in development aiming to modify the disease process itself by impacting one or more of the wide-ranging brain pathological changes that occur in individuals with the disease. These different approaches will target various sites where the disease begins and hopefully offer ways to prevent and/or slow AD's progression. Successful treatment may eventually involve a combination of medications aimed at several targets, similar to current state-of-the-art treatments for many cancers and AIDS (Alzheimer's Association, 2014h).

Beta-amyloid is being investigated, because it is the main component of plaques, a hallmark abnormality in the brain of an individual with AD. Scientists now have a detailed understanding of how this protein fragment is snipped from its parent amyloid precursor protein (APP) by two enzymes, beta-secretase and gamma-secretase. Researchers are developing medications aimed at virtually every point in this process of amyloid processing, including blocking activity of both enzymes, preventing the beta-amyloid fragments from clumping into plaques, and even using antibodies against beta-amyloid to clear it from the brain.

Tau protein is another area of investigation, as it is the main component of tangles, another brain abnormality hallmark in individuals with AD. Researchers are investigating strategies to keep these abnormal tau molecules from collapsing and twisting into tangles, a process that interferes with a vital cell transport system.

Inflammation is a potential target area to research, since it is another common brain abnormality in individuals with AD. Studies are investigating the body's overall inflammatory response to understand specific aspects of inflammation most active in the brain. This area of investigation may point to novel anti-inflammatory treatments for AD.

Insulin resistance and the way the brain cells process insulin may be linked to development of AD. Researchers are exploring the role of insulin in the brain and how brain cells utilize sugar (glucose) to produce energy. These investigations may reveal strategies to support cell function and put off Alzheimer's-related changes.

Assessing the Impact of Alzheimer's Disease on the Brain

Brain Imaging and Biomarkers. Many clinical trials using various brain imaging studies and laboratory testing of blood or spinal fluid are being conducted to provide methods to diagnose AD in its earliest, most treatable stages — possibly even before symptoms appear. Biomarkers are also being investigated, which may eventually offer improved methods to monitor the brain's response to treatment (Alzheimer's Association, 2014h).

Genetic/Familial Causes of Alzheimer Disease. The early-onset familial type of AD is an inherited form of the disease affecting individuals as young as 30 years. Investigations are being conducted on siblings of individuals who have early-onset AD and who have the genetic markers showing they will develop the disease. Experimental drugs are being studied in these individuals before symptoms begin to appear (Alzheimer's Association, 2014h).

Prevention Through Targeting Risk Factor Modification

There are several risk factors for developing AD, and a significant amount of research is being conducted to see if modifying these factors will prevent or slow the disease's progress (Weuve et al., 2014). The following are some of the primary risk factors for AD and descriptions of the research being done on each area:

- **Heavy Alcohol Use:** Some studies suggest an association between moderate alcohol consumption and a reduced risk of developing AD. Overall, data suggest that alcohol consumption is one of the modifiable factors that may have an impact on AD, with moderate use offering a minimal protective effect against developing the disease and heavy consumption promoting dementia, which may rapidly progress.

- **High Blood Pressure**: Maintaining blood pressure within normal, acceptable ranges (systolic below 140 and diastolic below 90; i.e., blood pressure below 140/90) may assist in diminishing risk of developing AD and slow the progression of the disease in the early stages. Cardiovascular disease and poorly controlled blood pressure readings may lead to more inflammation of the blood vessels and damage to brain cells caused by the inflamed vascular system. This inflammation leads to increased development of beta-amyloid proteins and incidence of the plaque of AD.

- **Diabetes Mellitus**: Controlling diabetes mellitus and managing insulin resistance, targeting hemoglobin A1c levels around 7% or less, offers some protection from developing AD and may slow the progression of the disease in the early stages. High levels of insulin in an individual with diabetes cause blood vessels to become inflamed. This inflammation sends off chemical markers which lead to tissue damage, with significant inflammation in the brain. One dangerous effect of this insulin-caused brain inflammation is increased brain levels of the beta-amyloid protein. As previously stated, beta-amyloid is the twisted protein that's the main ingredient of the sticky plaques that clog the brains of people with AD.

- **Head Injury**: Trauma to the brain has been shown as a risk factor for developing AD. This can be seen in individuals who have fallen and hit their head or have had blunt injury to the head (e.g., in football players, boxers, and individuals who have been in automobile accidents). Preventing head injury and protecting a person's head when he or she is at risk for it being hit is important. Research is being done on how individuals who sustain head injuries are more likely to develop AD. Studies are also examining preventive strategies to protect these individuals.

13

- **High Homocysteine Levels**: High homocysteine levels have been associated with an increased risk of developing AD. Current research is investigating ways to lower homocysteine levels. One area of study focuses on lowering levels through increased vitamin B intake.

- **Low Levels of Estrogen or Testosterone**: A 2007 study showed that women who used any form of estrogen therapy before age 65 were about 50% less likely to develop any form of dementia, including AD (Laino, 2007). However, most researchers agree that hormone replacement therapy does not protect women from diseases of aging, including AD, and taking these medications for long periods is associated with significant risks, including breast cancer, heart disease, and gall bladder disease (Steenhuysen, 2012). Regarding men, a recent study has uncovered a connection between testosterone and AD. A study at the National Institute on Aging (2004) found that men with AD had lower levels of free testosterone circulating in the bloodstream prior to being diagnosed. This has prompted researchers to study hormone replacement therapy with testosterone supplements in men.

- **Inflammation**: The development of inflammatory biomarkers for AD is being pursued, as this is essential to improve diagnosis and accelerate the development of new therapies. This line of research is imperative, since biochemical and neuroimaging markers can facilitate diagnosis and predict progression from a pre-AD state of mild cognitive impairment (MCI) to full-blown AD. These markers can also be used to monitor the efficacy of disease-modifying therapies (Chintamaneni & Bhaskar, 2012). It has been established that cerebrospinal fluid (CSF) levels of $A\beta40$, $A\beta42$, total tau, and phosphorylated tau have diagnostic value in assessing AD. Measurements of these CSF markers in combination are useful in predicting the risk of progression from MCI to AD. Expanding on this concept, new potential biomarkers are being identified, and CSF or plasma marker profiles may eventually

14

become part of a toolkit for accurate AD diagnosis and management. The ability to assess biomarkers along with clinical assessment, neuropsychological testing, and neuroimaging could result in more accurate in diagnosing AD and related disorders in the future.

- **Oxidative Stress**: In AD, oxidative stress plays a role in the degeneration of the brain. Diets high in certain antioxidants have been found to be protective against the disease. An entire chapter is devoted to discussing dietary and other lifestyle strategies for preventing and slowing the disease (see Chapter 6).

- **Obesity**: A recent study has suggested that today's obesity epidemic may be tomorrow's AD epidemic. It has been noted that people with diabetes are at a higher risk of developing AD, but there is now strong evidence that people with high insulin levels are on the road to developing AD long before they are clinically diagnosed with diabetes. As the body becomes more and more overweight, it becomes more resistant to the blood sugar–lowering effects of insulin. To counter this resistance, the body makes more insulin, and as this process continues, the escalating cycle of insulin resistance and insulin production ends in a clinical presentation of diabetes mellitus type 2 (Craft, 2009; DeNoon, 2005). High levels of insulin cause blood vessels to become inflamed, which sends off chemical markers that initiate a cascade of events leading to tissue damage, including inflammation in the brain. One dangerous effect of insulin-caused brain inflammation is increased brain levels of the beta-amyloid protein, the main ingredient of the sticky plaques that clog the brain in AD.

- **Low Physical Activity**: Physical activity increases blood flow and oxygenation to body tissues, including the brain. It has also been shown to decrease insulin resistance, which, as previously discussed, is a significant factor in development of AD. Although a combination of diet and

15

physical activity has been shown to slow the development of AD, increasing physical activity alone was shown to significantly decrease the incidence AD (Scarmeas et al., 2009). A more in-depth discussion of physical activity is presented in Chapters 6 and 7.

Chapter 2

MILD COGNITIVE IMPAIRMENT

Mild cognitive impairment (MCI) can be the beginning of AD, as well as other forms of dementia in an older person. This chapter discusses the pathophysiology of MCI and how the symptoms present in an elder.

Where are the keys? We looked all over the house, unable to find the car keys. Mom actually had "back-up" keys, because this happened fairly frequently. Misplacing car keys is not an uncommon problem for many older people, but putting the car keys in odd places such as the freezer may indicate there is a more serious problem. The freezer is where we found Mom's car keys, and it was on that day when I began to wonder if there was something wrong.

Mild cognitive impairment is defined as deficits in an individual's memory that do not significantly impact his or her daily functioning abilities (UCSF Memory and Aging Center, 2013). These memory problems may be minimal to mild and hardly noticeable by the individual. An older person may start using memory triggers to compensate for these mild cognitive problems, such as using written notes or reminders and keeping logs. Unlike AD, in which cognitive abilities progressively decline, MCI results in memory deficits that may remain stable for years. However, some individuals with MCI develop cognitive deficits and functional impairment consistent with AD. MCI has been referred to as a transitional zone between normal aging and dementia (Raschetti et al., 2007).

In addition to memory problems, MCI causes a slight decline in other cognitive skills, such as reasoning abilities. Studies suggest that 10 to 20% of those older than 65 have some degree of MCI. MCI causes changes that may be serious enough to be noticed by the individuals experiencing them or to other people, but they are not severe enough to interfere with the ability to live independently or to perform the usual activities of daily living. A person with MCI does not usually meet diagnostic criteria for dementia. In older individuals, certain symptoms of MCI can be caused by other factors or conditions, such as an infection (e.g., urinary tract infection, upper respiratory infection), medications (e.g., pain medications, anxiety medications), stress, audio and/or visual overstimulation, dehydration, or other conditions (e.g., anemia, bradycardia [slow heart rate]). Any older person with symptoms of MCI should seek a medical evaluation to rule out a treatable (and reversible) cause. However, those with true MCI do have an increased risk of eventually developing AD or another type of dementia (Alzheimer's Association, 2014e).

Symptoms

In individuals with MCI, memory complaints typically include difficulty remembering the names of people they have recently met, difficulty remembering the flow of a conversation (i.e., losing one's train of thought), and an increased tendency to misplace things. Often, the person will be aware of these problems and able to compensate with increased reliance on notes and calendars (USCF Memory and Aging Center, n.d.). These problems are similar to but less severe than those in AD. There are two types of MCI: amnesiac and nonamnesiac (Peterson, 2011):

- **Amnesiac MCI:** The person may forget important information that would previously have been easy to recall, such as appointments, conversations, or recent events.

- **Nonamnesiac MCI:** The person has impairments in thinking skills that affect the ability to make sound decisions, judge time or sequence of steps needed to complete a complex task, or visual perception.

Medical Work-Up

The medical evaluation for someone with symptoms of MCI should include a thorough exploration of the memory complaints, including a discussion of what the actual symptoms are, the type of information being forgotten and when (e.g., time of day, when stressed), the duration of the problem (over what period of time, if the symptoms are worsening), and whether other cognitive complaints are occurring (e.g., problems with organization, planning, visual-spatial abilities). The following should also be included in the work-up (Alzheimer's Association, n.d.):

- **Medical history**: Current symptoms and their history of the onset; previous medical conditions; recent illnesses; history of confusion experienced in the past; family history of significant memory problems or dementia, including AD; vital signs; list of medications used; use of alcohol, tobacco, caffeine, and any street drugs; and history of falls.

- **Assessment of independent function and daily activities**: Ability to perform Activities of Daily Living (ADLs), which include basic activities (e.g. eating, bathing, dressing, toileting, transferring (walking), and continence), and Instrumental Activities of Daily Living (IADLs), which include abilities that allow a person to live independently (e.g., ability to use telephone, shop, prepare meals, clean the house, do laundry, drive a vehicle, manage medications [remember what to take and how often], and manage finances).

- **Information about cognitive abilities from family or friends**: Additional information on cognition and ability to function in day-to-day activities; perspectives on how an individual's function may have changed.

- **Assessment of mental status**: Brief tests to evaluate memory (recent as well as remote [long-term]), planning abilities, judgment, ability to follow simple instructions,

19

ability to understand visual information, and other key thinking skills.

- **Medical evaluation, including a neurological examination**: Full medical evaluation to determine health status and assess the function of nerves and reflexes, movement, gait (ambulation/walking), coordination, balance, and senses (i.e., vision, hearing, smell, taste, touch).

- **Psychological evaluation**: Basic evaluation of the individual's mood and personality to detect depression and/or anxiety and assess symptoms such as problems with memory or feeling "spacey" or "foggy."

- **Medication causes of memory problems**: Medications used by older individuals that may impair memory, such as anxiety medications (benzodiazepines; e.g., Ativan, Xanax, Valium), diphenhydramine (Benadryl, Tylenol PM, Advil PM, etc.), benztropine (Cogentin), oxybutinon (Detrol, Ditropan), and many others.

- **Laboratory tests**: Blood tests to rule out other medical conditions that could affect memory, such as anemia, including complete blood count (CBC); tests of electrolyte imbalances, kidney function, and liver function (Complete Metabolic Panel); thyroid panel; tests for HIV; rapid plasma reagin test (RPR, for syphilis); urinalysis; and possibly imaging of the brain's structure. Consider additional screenings, such as for drug use, lead, mercury, ammonia levels, and vitamin B and D levels.

This type of work-up may identify other health issues causing the cognitive impairment, but if it does not create a clear clinical picture, neuropsychological testing may be recommended, which involves a series of written or computerized tests to evaluate specific thinking skills administered by an expert at this type of evaluation.

Progression

Mild cognitive impairment may or may not progress to AD. There are certain features of cognitive impairment that have been associated with a higher likelihood of progressing to full AD. These include a person's memory impairment being reported by a family member or friend rather than by the individual, poor performance on objective memory testing, and any changes in the ability to perform daily tasks (e.g., housekeeping, laundry, driving, medication management, or financial management), difficulty handling a tough situation or an emergency, or a decline in a person's ability to maintain personal hygiene (UCSF Memory and Aging Center, 2013).

Treatment

Currently there are no specific treatments for MCI. Essentially, the most appropriate plan of care would be monitoring the affected person's medical and psychological health and watching for changes in condition and/or function. Some health care practitioners encourage the use of medical interventions that were designed for use in AD, such as cholinesterase inhibitors (donepezil, rivastigmine, galantamine). However, because most studies are inconclusive about whether MCI progresses to AD, there is no clear and convincing evidence to support the use of cholinesterase inhibitors or any other treatments for the disorder. Researchers are still determining whether data from trials in individuals with MCI or AD indicate any beneficial effects of medication in slowing cognitive decline. There is strong evidence to suggest that recognizing MCI and early symptoms of AD as early as possible is important to increase the potential for early treatment, which is the best way to slow the destruction of the plaques and tangles of AD (USCF Memory and Aging Center, n.d.).

As stated, although not indicated or approved to treat MCI, three cholinesterase inhibitors are commonly prescribed in certain individuals in whom the diagnosis of MCI versus early AD is unclear. These are as follows:

- Donepezil (Aricept), which is approved to treat all stages of AD.

- Rivastigmine (Exelon), which is approved to treat mild to moderate AD.

- Galantamine (Razadyne), which is approved to treat mild to moderate AD.

Treating Other Conditions That May Affect Mental Function

Being forgetful or less mentally sharp than usual may be misdiagnosed as MCI in some older individuals. Identifying and managing other medical conditions may help improve a person's memory and overall mental function. The following are conditions that can affect memory:

- **Hypertension:** High blood pressure that is poorly controlled can worsen problems with memory and cognitive functioning.

- **Hypotension:** Low blood pressure can cause cognition and memory problems.

- Bradycardia: When the heart rate is too slow to adequately profuse the brain with blood and oxygen, the person may be confused and have problems with cognition.

- **Anemia:** When hemoglobin and hematocrit levels are too low and there are not enough blood cells to transport oxygen to the brain, a person may be confused and have issues with cognition.

- **Depression:** When a person is depressed, sometimes he or she becomes forgetful and mentally dull. Depression is common in people with MCI. Treating depression may help improve memory and make it easier to cope with the changes in life.

- **Anxiety:** Anxiety can cause a person to be less aware of his or her surroundings, appear confused, and have problems with memory and cognition. Managing anxiety may improve an individual's cognitive abilities.
- **Sleep apnea:** Sleep apnea results in breathing being repeatedly interrupted: Periods of cessation of respiration are followed by the abrupt restarting of breathing during sleep, making it difficult for the person to get a good night's rest. During these periods of respiration cessation, the brain suffers from lack of oxygenation (hypoxia), which can lead to worsening of high blood pressure and other medical conditions. Sleep apnea can also make a person feel fatigued during the day, forgetful, and unable to concentrate and may worsen other cognitive abilities. Treatment can improve these symptoms and restore alertness. A medical evaluation is important to manage this problem.

CHAPTER 3

DIAGNOSING AND
TREATING ALZHEIMER'S DISEASE

THIS CHAPTER DISCUSSES THE PATHOPHYSIOLOGY OF AD, RISK FACTORS FOR DEVELOPING THE DISORDER, PRESENTING SYMPTOMS, HOW TO DIAGNOSE AD, AND CURRENT TREATMENTS.

Mom did not believe that she could pay all the bills, so she decided to not pay any of them. Her reasoning was that she would die soon, so "why bother." When Mom told me about the foreclosure notice on her home and we began to look into the issue, we discovered the problem was much bigger than any of the family knew. Forgetting to pay a bill or forgetting to pick up milk while at the grocery store may be common for any older person, but being unable to manage finances and think logically indicates a much bigger issue. There was enough income to cover the bills, and Mom had managed her financial affairs for years, but she could no longer manage her personal affairs due to cognitive impairment affecting her executive functioning (which she did not realize was diminishing). She was a smart woman who helped anyone who needed help; she even helped her sister when needed, after her divorce, helping her find a job, buy a house, and establish a monthly budget. But now, Mom could no longer even manage her monthly bills, believing there wasn't enough money to pay for everything.

Normal Brain Functioning

The brain is the control center for the body. Physiologically, the brain exerts control over every bodily system. The brain acts to coordinate the rest of the body, by both generating movement or muscle activity and driving secretion of chemicals that affect the body's systems. This centralized control system allows rapid and coordinated responses to stimulation from the environment. There are some basic types of responsiveness, such as reflexes, which are mediated by the spinal cord, but sophisticated purposeful control of movement and behavior is based on complex sensory input requiring the information-integrating capabilities of the brain. The brain performs an incredible number of tasks, including controlling basic body functions (body temperature, blood pressure, heart rate, and breathing), accepting information about an individual's surroundings from various senses (seeing, hearing, smelling, tasting, and touching), coordinating physical movement (walking, talking, standing, or sitting), and allowing a person to think, dream, reason, and experience emotions.

The most basic working unit in the brain is the neuron, which is the signaling unit of the nervous system, and the human brain contains billions. The neurons' interactions with one another enable a person to think, move, maintain balance, and feel emotions. These specialized cells produce different actions because of their precise connections with other neurons, sensory receptors, and muscle cells (National Institutes of Health, 2010). A typical neuron has three primary parts: the cell body, dendrites, and axons. Information is conveyed from one neuron to another by using electrical and chemical signals.

When a neuron is triggered, it creates an internal signal for action (e.g., to store information, to think, to make muscles move). Once the neuron is triggered, an electrical impulse travels the length of the neuron, and at the end of the neuron a chemical is released to communicate with the next neuron and continues on to multiple neurons until the action occurs. Neurons' ability to communicate with one another is very fast; thus, movements and actions occur almost instantaneously if the neurons are intact and the chemicals within the brain are in proper balance.

Changes to the Brain in Alzheimer's Disease

Alzheimer's disease causes physiological changes in the brain and eventually leads to reduced physical functioning. However, the majority of symptoms are presented psychologically (e.g., declines in memory and ability to reason, mood and personality changes). The physiological, or structural, changes occurring in the brain include development of plaques (between the neurons) and tangles (within the neuron/nerve cells) as well as chemical imbalances in the neurotransmitters (acetylcholine, glutamate, serotonin, and dopamine). AD usually begins slowly and progresses over time, causing worsening of the symptoms. In an individual with AD, changes within the brain include shriveling of the cortex; damage to areas involved in thinking, planning and remembering; shrinkage of brain size, more severe in the hippocampus, an area of the cortex that plays a key role in formation of new memories; and growth of the ventricles (chambers within the brain containing cerebrospinal fluid).

Plaques and Tangles

As mentioned previously, myloid plaques develop between nerve cells (neurons) in the brain with AD. Amyloids are naturally occurring within the brain — they are protein fragments that the body produces. Beta-amyloid is a fragment of these proteins, which are clipped from another protein called APP. In an individual with a healthy brain, these proteins occur normally. The fragments break down and are then eliminated in a controlled manner. In a person with AD, the fragments are not disposed of properly and begin to accumulate to form hard, insoluble plaques.

Another feature in the brain with AD is neurofibrillary tangles. As discussed in previous chapters, these are insoluble twisted fibers found within the brain's nerve cells. Tau is a protein that forms the microtubules, structures responsible for transporting nutrients and other important substances from one part of the nerve cell to another. Tangles primarily consist of these tau proteins. In a person with AD, the tau protein is abnormal, and the microtubule structures are not functioning properly, collapsing and causing problems with the conduction of brain cell nerve impulses (Bright Focus Foundation, 2013).

As the disease progresses, the brain tissue shrinks, and the ventricles become enlarged. In the early stages of AD, the brain cells in the hippocampus begin to degenerate, leading to short-term memory impairment and declines in recent memory. Cell destruction spreads through the brain, progressing toward the cerebral cortex (the outer layer of the brain), leading to problems in logical thinking abilities and judgment, emotional outbursts, and language impairment. The disease usually continues to advance throughout the brain, leading to the death of more nerve cells, with subsequent changes in behavior, such as erratic actions, wandering, and possibly agitation. In the final stages of AD, an individual may lose the ability to perform basic ADLs, such as the ability to feed him- or herself, speak, recognize people, and control bodily functions (Bright Focus Foundation, 2013).

Chemical Imbalances

There are four chemicals that become out of balance in individuals with AD: acetylcholine, glutamate, serotonin, and dopamine (Chen et al., 2011). *Acetylcholine* is a neurotransmitter that helps transmit nerve impulses to muscle cells, signaling them to contract. Too little acetylcholine is seen in the brain of individuals with AD, but acetylcholine imbalances can also be seen in people with Parkinson's disease and or multiple sclerosis. As previously mentioned, in 1906, a German scientist named Alois Alzheimer treated a patient with an atypical form of dementia, previously referred to as *old age dementia*. When the patient died, Dr. Alzheimer performed an autopsy and found that her acetylcholine pathways were severely damaged by neurofibrillary tangles, and her brain had an excess of plaque. In AD, acetylcholine is the first chemical neurotransmitter affected — it is destroyed too rapidly and is not available to allow the neurons to communicate with one another.

Glutamate is another neurotransmitter that is a type of amino acid. Glutamate is the main inhibitory neurotransmitter of the central nervous system. It plays a role in regulating neuronal excitability throughout the nervous system and is directly responsible for the regulation of muscle tone. In the middle stage of AD, glutamate is produced more rapidly, resulting in an excess in the brain. This causes the affected person to be more easily excited and agitated and can lead to verbal outbursts and erratic behaviors.

Serotonin is a monoamine neurotransmitter that is believed to play a role in person's sense of well-being and happiness. Serotonin also affects the regulation of mood, appetite, and sleep. Serotonin does impact some cognitive functions, including memory and learning. In AD, serotonin is not as readily available, causing increased mood swings. Several classes of pharmacological antidepressants, the selective serotonin reuptake inhibitors (SSRIs), modulate serotonin.

Dopamine is the final chemical impacted in AD. In the brain, dopamine functions as a neurotransmitter involved in motor control and controlling the release of several important hormones. Dopamine is also involved in the regulation of cognitive processes. Dopamine is closely associated with serotonin, and in individuals with AD, both neurotransmitters influence the non-cognitive symptoms of the disease that impair daily living, such as anxiety, depression, apathy, and psychosis. Researchers believe the level of dopamine may be low in people with AD.

Memory Impairment

As has been discussed, memory impairment in AD progresses from short-term (recent) to long-term (remote) memories. In some individuals, memories may become almost nonexistent. It has been noted that the younger an individual is when he or she begins exhibiting the symptoms of AD, the faster the progression. However, the rate of progression depends on the type of AD the individual has. (The different types of AD are discussed later in this chapter.) On average, people with AD live for 8 to 10 years after diagnosis. Some individuals survive as long as 20 years, but AD is a terminal disease, as it leads to the bodily systems shutting down in the final stages ("Bright Focus Foundation," 2013). There are many factors that can hasten the progression of the disease, as well as others that can slow it down. For example, general anesthesia has been linked to exacerbation of the progression of AD in the early stages of disease (i.e., AD progresses at a faster pace within the initial 6 months following the use of general anesthesia; Kapoor, 2011). Lifestyle factors can slow the disease progression. Later in this book, ways to slow the progression through diet, exercise (both physical and brain exercises), and environment are presented.

Physical Changes of Alzheimer's Disease

As mentioned in prior sections, in AD, plaques develop within the brain, beginning in the hippocampus, a structure deep in the brain that helps store memories. The plaques progress toward other areas of the brain, initially to the cerebral cortex, which influences a person's ability to think and make decisions (Anderson, 2014). There are also tangles and chemical imbalances. These are the major hallmarks of AD in the brain (National Institute on Aging, 2012). Following is a review of these phenomena:

- **Amyloid plaques**: Made up of fragments of a protein called beta-amyloid peptide mixed with a collection of additional proteins, remnants of neurons, and pieces of other nerve cells.

- **Neurofibrillary tangles**: Found inside neurons; abnormal collections of a protein called tau. Normal tau is required for a healthy neuron. However, in AD, tau clumps together, causing the neurons to be unable to function normally; this eventually causes the neurons to die.

- **Loss of connections between neurons responsible for memory and learning**: Neurons must communicate to function and survive; when they lose their connections to other neurons, they die. As neurons die throughout the brain, the affected areas begin to atrophy, or shrink. By the final stage of AD, damage is widespread, and the entire brain has shrunken significantly.

• **Chemical imbalances**: Neurons require chemicals (neurotransmitters) to communicate with other neurons to allow proper brain functioning. As plaques and tangles form, the brain chemicals become out of balance, which impairs the neurons' ability to communicate with one another. As previously stated, the four chemicals that are mainly affected are acetylcholine, glutamate, serotonin, and dopamine.

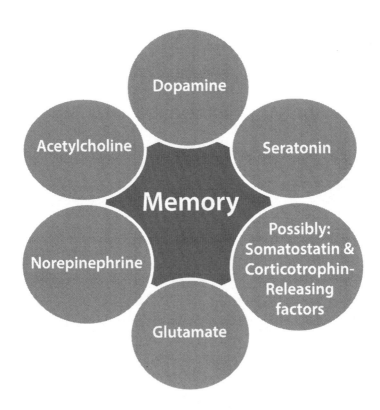

How Does Alzheimer's Disease Progress?

The progression of Alzheimer's disease has been briefly outlined in previous sections. This section provides more details about the stages of disease and how cognitive and other functions are affected.

As noted, MCI can present with symptoms similar to those of the early stages of AD and causes more memory problems than normal for people of the same age. Many, but not all, individuals with MCI will develop AD (NIND, 2013). Despite a significant amount of research being conducted to identify the factors causing AD to progress more rapidly and ways to halt the progression of the disease process, no treatment has yet been identified to stop the disease. However, some medications help slow the progression of AD and keep symptoms from getting worse for a period of time (National Institutes of Health, 2013). This will help people with AD stay more independent and lessen the impact on the caregiver. Some keys things to remember about the progression of AD are as follow:

- Symptoms vary from person to person — some symptoms appear earlier or later than indicated here, or not at all.

- Stages may overlap — an individual may be unable to do certain things, may need help with one task, or may be able to manage another activity independently.

- Some symptoms may appear at one point and then vanish, while others, such as memory loss, will worsen over time.

Each person with AD will have a different course of the disease, and this will depend on many factors, including genetic make-up, other medical conditions, activity level, diet, emotional resilience, medications, and support system. The life expectancy of an individual with AD will also vary, depending on the age when he or she got the disease, but is on average 8 to 10 years. In general, someone who develops AD after age 60, could experience a progression of the disease over 8 to 20 years from the time of diagnosis (Alzheimer's Association, 2014i; Byrd, 2011), whereas someone diagnosed in his or her 90s may live for about 3-5 years. Those who develop "early-onset AD" may have a life expectancy of 5 to 8 years after the start of symptoms. Life expectancy also depends on how early in the process the diagnosis was made, as well as the treatment plan (Alzheimer's Association, 2014j).

Following is a description of typical symptoms at each stage of the disease.

Early Stage

Alzheimer's disease begins gradually with very minor changes in the person's abilities or behavior. In some individuals, these signs may be mistaken for normal aging changes or due to stress. Sometimes these symptoms are only noticed after the fact. Loss of memory for recent events is a common early sign. A person in the early stages of AD may also experience the following:

- Begins to forget conversations, information related to other people, recent events
- Has decreased attention span
- Is less motivated to complete tasks
- Gets lost in familiar places
- Problems with language: Repeats same words or stories over and over, uses substitute or rhyming words
- Forgets names and words; may make up words or stories to fill in memory gaps
- Misplaces things or puts them in strange locations
- Develops a tendency to blame others for taking mislaid items
- Trouble with abstract thinking: begins to think concretely
- Becomes slower at grasping new ideas
- Becomes unable to follow a series of instructions
- Becomes confused at times

- Shows poor judgment
- Finds it difficult to make decisions
- Loses interest in events, as well as other people or activities
- Becomes unwilling to try out new things and has difficulty adapting to change
- Changes in mood: Becomes depressed, irritable, or anxious
- Is more quick to anger and frustration, gets tired easily, feels rushed, is more easily surprised
- Becomes insensitive to others' feelings
- Begins to exhibit idiosyncratic behavior (e.g., hoarding, checking behavior, searching for objects with little obvious value)
- Forgets to eat or eats constantly

Middle or Moderate Stage

As AD progresses, the changes become more marked. The individual may require assistance with managing day-to-day activities. He or she may need reminders or assistance to eat, wash, dress, and use the toilet. The person will become increasingly forgetful, particularly of names, and may repeat him- or herself, asking the same question or saying the same phrase over and over. The individual may also fail to recognize people or confuse them with others. Symptoms may include:

- Having poor short-term memory, forgetting recent history
- Having more difficulty with names and faces of friends and family: May remember people as they were 10–20 years ago, may be able to distinguish familiar from unfamiliar but may not remember specifics of individuals
- Knowing own name and date of birth but possibly forgetting own age

- Becoming confused about where he or she is, forgetting current or most recent address and phone number
- Wandering off and becoming lost
- Becoming disoriented and confused about time (e.g., season, day of week, time of day)
- Getting days and nights mixed up (e.g., getting up at night, sleeping during the day)
- Inability to think logically, tendency to be difficult to reason with, it becomes difficult to explain things to him or her in a logical way
- Inability to organize own speech or thoughts, difficulty following the logic of others, having flight of ideas
- Inability to follow written or oral instructions or sequence of steps (e.g., recipes), inability to read lengthy articles or other materials
- Inability to add and subtract, leading to math and financial difficulties
- Putting him- or herself or others at risk through forgetfulness
  » By turning the gas on but not lighting the stove
  » By not paying attention to traffic while driving

- Behaving in ways that seem unusual, such as wearing a shirt inside-out
- Experiencing difficulty with sensory perception, having hallucinations
- Becoming easily upset, angry, or aggressive
- Losing his or her confidence and becoming very dependent or clingy

Late Stage

During this stage, the person with AD eventually becomes totally dependent on others for all care. Loss of memory becomes pronounced, and the person is unable to perform the most basic tasks, such as eating and swallowing and recognizing the need to urinate. The person will be unable to recognize familiar objects or surroundings, although there may be sudden flashes of recognition. The individual may begin having difficulty with mobility, shuffling or walking unsteadily, eventually becoming confined to bed or a wheelchair. Other symptoms may include the following:

- Continued decline of mental/cognitive abilities
- Deterioration of personality: May become withdrawn or more aggressive
- Becoming distressed or aggressive, especially if feeling threatened in any way; may have angry outbursts, such as during close personal care because the person does not understand what is happening
- Physical problems begin: May not recognize thirst or hunger, may have difficulty with eating and swallowing (increased choking), may not recognize need to use bathroom or shift positions
- Deterioration of voluntary control of bodily functions and mobility (losing control of bladder function and bowels, inability to walk)
- Pocketing or holding in mouth of food or medications
- Considerable weight loss, although some people eat too much and gain weight
- Gradual loss of speech, although the person may speak incoherently, repeat a few words, cry out from time to time, or ramble; loss of ability to express emotions appropriately, loss of ability to smile
- Restlessness, sometimes seeming to be searching for someone or something; may seem uncomfortable and cry when touched or moved

- Inability to write or read, seeming to have little understanding of speech and not recognizing those around him or her
  - » The person may still respond to affection and to being talked to in a calm and soothing voice
  - » The person may also enjoy scents, music, or stroking a pet or stuffed animal

Terminal Stage

In the final stage of AD, the person is dependent for all activities of daily living: moving, eating, and toileting. The person is unable to hold his or her body weight upright and becomes chair- or bedbound, is less mobile, and loses weight. As the disease progresses, the individual's immune system begins to fail, and he or she may experience respiratory infections and/or urinary tract infections. Eventually, the person cannot fight off these infections or experiences other complications that lead to death. The following symptoms are common:

- Inability to remember the sequence of eating, including swallowing, inability to swallow (increased incidence of choking/aspiration)
- Decreased respiratory efforts
  - » Increased respiratory infections
- Decreased ability to move trunk and extremities
  - » Inability to sit upright on own, may "scoot" in chair
  - » Muscle atrophy/weight loss
  - » Becoming contracted in fetal position
  - » Increased incidence of pressure ulcers
- Incontinent of urine and feces
  - » Increased incidence of urinary tract infections
  - » Increased incidence of constipation/fecal impactions
- Failure of immune system
  - » Recurrent urinary tract infections
  - » Recurrent pneumonias
- Death

Diagnosing Alzheimer's Disease

In any individual in whom AD is suspected, a full medical work-up is necessary to rule out other conditions (see Table 3-1). A diagnosis of AD is often made based on presentation of symptoms, findings on neurologic examination, and results from diagnostic tests (Mayo Clinic, 2014b). Certain forms of AD can be detected through laboratory tests, and early-onset AD, also known as the familial form, can be identified through DNA testing. However, other forms of AD, the later-onset types, do not have blood markers. Certain individuals can be diagnosed with magnetic resonance imaging (MRI) testing when there is a significant atrophy of the hippocampus, but this atrophy can be difficult to identify, as it may be so slight that it is not readily noticed (Ramachandran, 2013). There are not yet guidelines or recommendations for the standardized use of MRI.

Initially, any individual who presents with confusion should have a complete physical exam, including laboratory tests and a detailed history of symptoms, medical issues, medications, recent injuries/falls, and surgeries. Examination by a neurology specialist may be done to assist in ruling out other conditions, such as Parkinson's disease, strokes, tumors, and other medical conditions that may impair memory and thinking, as well as physical function.

Table 3-1. Diagnosing Alzheimer's Disease
• Person's medical and psychiatric history; may get some information from family, friends, and caregivers
• Information about the main problem, including any symptoms of confusion or difficulty in day-to-day functioning
• Information about other symptoms
• Medical history, including whether the person has a history of falling
• Medications, both prescription and over the counter
• Psychosocial history: Marital status, living conditions, employment, sexual history, important life events
• Mental state: Any evidence of psychiatric problems, such as depression, anxiety, or memory impairment
• Family history, including any illnesses that run in the family

Laboratory Tests

The laboratory tests employed in a standard work-up are intended to rule out other causes of dementia, such as electrolyte imbalances, nutritional deficiencies, infection, drug effects, and other conditions. Common tests include the following:

- Urinalysis and microscopy
- CBC to rule out anemia and infection
- Serum electrolyte levels to identify metabolic disease
- Serum chemistry panel, including liver function tests
- Thyroid panel to rule out hypothyroidism
- Serum vitamin B12 test to rule out deficiency
- Serum vitamin D test to rule out deficiency
- Neurosyphilis serology to rule out syphilis
- Urine toxicology to rule out medication/drug use

- Serum toxicology (for alcohol, medications, drugs, and other substances)
- Erythrocyte sedimentation rate to screen for connective tissue disease
- HIV titer to rule out HIV/AIDS

Risk Factors for Developing Alzheimer's Disease

When conducting a work-up in an individual with possible symptoms of AD, the following are considered risk factors (University of Maryland Medical Center, 2012).

- Age is the greatest risk factor for AD. Most individuals who develop AD are older than 65 years, and the risk increases with age. People 85 years and older are especially at risk.

- Gender: More women than men develop AD, but this risk factor is not clearly understood; there are more older women than men, since historically women tend to live longer.

- Race and ethnicity: African Americans and Hispanics are at greater risk for developing AD than are non-Hispanic white individuals. This could be due to the fact that African American and Hispanics have a higher prevalence of medical conditions such as high blood pressure and diabetes that are associated with increased risk for Alzheimer's.

- Family history: People with a family history of AD are at higher than average risk for the disease.

- Heart and vascular diseases: Researchers are currently investigating whether diseases that affect the heart and vascular system may increase the risk for AD. These conditions include high blood pressure, unhealthy cholesterol levels, and type 2 diabetes. There is some evidence suggesting that controlling these conditions may help prevent AD.

Neuropsychological Testing

Neuropsychological testing studies an individual's behavior and mood and attempts to clarify the type of dementia an individual has when confusion presents. It is utilized when a person is having significant problems with memory, concentration, understanding, visual-spatial issues, and a variety of other symptoms. It is useful in differentiating between AD and psychiatric problems such as depression and anxiety, problems caused by medications, issues of substance abuse, strokes, and tumors. Neuropsychological testing is a lengthy process administered over an average of 8 hours and includes a comprehensive interview with the person and tests to assess memory, language, the ability to plan and reason, and the ability to modify behavior, as well as assessments of personality and emotional stability (Chapman et al., 2010).

- Neuropsychological tests are required for a more definitive clinical diagnosis of Alzheimer's
- They are helpful for ruling out other types of dementia
- They enable the healthcare provider to document the progression of the disease
- They can identify depression or suicidal ideation, which can be treated

Mini-Mental State Exam

The Mini-Mental State Examination (MMSE), developed by Drs. Marshal Folstein and Susan Folstein, offers a quick and simple way to get an estimate of cognitive abilities and screen for cognitive loss. It is not a diagnostic test but a test that assesses the progression of cognitive function and its decline over time. It can assist with measuring the progression of AD in an individual when the test is administered periodically and scores are compared to show improvement in cognition, stabilization in cognition, or decline in cognition. It tests the person's orientation, attention, calculation, recall, language, and motor skills.

41

Each section of the MMSE involves a series of questions or commands. The individual receives one point for each correct answer. The administrator of the test is seated with the person in a quiet, well-lit room. The individual is asked to listen carefully and answer each question as accurately as he or she can. The test is not timed, and the scoring is immediate. The maximum score is 30 points. In general, a score between 25 and 30 indicates adequate cognitive functioning; scores between 24 and 20 indicate mild cognitive impairment; between 19 and 10 indicates moderate cognitive impairment; and a score below 10 indicates severe cognitive impairment. The raw score may need to be corrected for educational level and age. Low scores may indicate the presence of dementia, although other mental disorders can lead to abnormal findings. Physical problems can also interfere with interpretation if not properly noted; for example, an individual being unable to hear or read instructions properly or having a motor deficit that affects writing and drawing skills may cause the scores to be abnormally low ("Mini-Mental State Exam," n.d.). Despite the many free versions of the test that are available on the Internet, the official version is copyrighted and must be ordered through Psychological Assessment Resources (PAR).

Clock Drawing Test

The Clock Drawing Test (CDT) is a simple test that can be used as a part of a neurological test or as a simple screening tool for Alzheimer's and other types of dementia. The test can provide information about general cognitive and adaptive functioning, such as memory, processing information, and visual-spatial issues It is highly correlated with the MMSE, and a normal clock drawing almost always correlates with normal cognitive abilities (Kennard, 2006).

Clock Drawing Test

Draw a clock with face

Tell the person to put a specific time on the clock; i.e., 2:30

Provide paper and a writing utensil

<u>Scoring</u>

1 point for the clock circle

1 point for all the numbers being in the correct order

1 point for the numbers being in the proper spatial arrangement

1 point for the two hands of the clock

1 point for the correct time

MAXIMUM SCORE = 5 POINTS

OR

Tell patient to draw a clock with the time at 11:10

10 point scoring (1 point each):

a) 12 in correct location   1 point

b) 1 and 2 in correct location   2 points

c) 7, 8, 10, 11 in correct location   4 points

d) 1, 2, 4, 5, 7, 8, 10, 11 in correct location   8 points

*no points for hands of clock if same length, no matter their position

e) 1, 2, 4, 5, 7, 8, 10, 11 in correct location   8 points

Little hand on 11 = 1 point; big hand on 2 = 1 point (total 10 points)

Mini-Cog Test

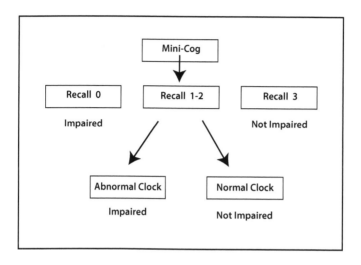

The Mini-Cog is a quick and easy test that takes about 3 minutes to administer and is often used to assist in identifying people who require further investigation into their clinical presentation. The test consists of a three-item recall and a clock drawing test. First, the person is asked to remember three items and then is asked to draw a clock (the same as in the CDT). Then the person is then asked to recall the three words. If he or she is unable to recall three words, some form of dementia is present; if able to name one or two words and able to perform an adequate CDT, then dementia of Alzheimer's disease is probably not present; if able to name one or two words and unable to perform an adequate CDT, then there is probably some form of dementia present; and if the individual is able to recall all three items, he or she probably does not have dementia, depending on other symptoms (Kennard, 2006).

Differential Diagnosis

Alzheimer's disease is the most common form of dementia in individuals older than 65 years and accounts for up to 80% of all dementia cases. When attempting to develop a diagnosis, other forms of dementia must be ruled out, because they may have symptoms and pathologies similar to AD. Knowing the key features and pathology of each type of dementia can help in accurate diagnosis, to ensure that people receive the treatment and support services appropriate for their condition and help them maintain the highest possible quality of life. The following list details the symptoms of AD compared with those of other forms of dementia:

- **AD**: Hallmark symptom is the slow or insidious onset of symptoms, usually beginning with an inability to remember new information. May be associated with early impairment in language and visual-spatial or executive function. The individual usually has a normal neurological exam. Brain images show increased hippocampal and overall brain atrophy, but absolute levels of shrinkage have not yet been quantified and standardized. There is growing evidence suggesting that with advancing age, dementia that "looks like" Alzheimer's is probably due to a combination of AD pathology and other disorders, known as "mixed dementia."

- **MCI**: An individual may report having intermittent difficulties with memory and slight confusion in certain situations that do not cause significant impact on daily functioning. Memory deficits appear to be relative to norms for age and education and are objectively evident on a mental status exam or neuropsychological testing. Cognition is essentially normal.

- **Vascular dementia**: This is the second most common cause of dementia, accounting for about 20 to 30% of all cases. The clinical picture may be impairment in one or more cognitive domains within a few months after a stroke. This condition is sometimes called *post-stroke dementia*. Specific cognitive domains affected depend on the location of the stroke. Problems in attention and executive function are common. Memory loss may or may not be prominent, depending on whether the stroke affected memory areas. The cognitive problem depends on the size of the stroke: If a large area was affected, then a sudden cognitive problem will be evident. If the stroke is microscopic and numerous small strokes occur, the cognitive problems may have a slow onset, in a stepwise approach. The individual may have risk factors for vascular disease, such as a history of high blood pressure, elevated lipids, diabetes, or past heart attacks or strokes. "Pure" vascular dementia may be relatively unusual; vascular changes may more commonly co-exist with Alzheimer's plaques or other forms of dementia. The Hachinski Ischemic Scale (HIS) is a tool widely used to identify a likely vascular component once a dementia diagnosis has been established. A shortened seven-item version of the HIS has been validated. A score ≤ 2 suggests vascular involvement (Hachinski et al., 2012).

Table 3-2. Reduced Seven-Item Hachinkski Ischemic Score		
Item Description	**Yes**	**No**
Abrupt onset		
Stepwise deterioration		
Fluctuating course		
Emotional incontinence		
History of stroke		
Focal neurological symptoms		
Focal neurological signs		
Total "Yes" Answers		
From Hachinski et al. (2012)		

- **Mixed dementia**: As stated, when an individual has more than one form of dementia, such as AD and vascular dementia coexisting, it is known as mixed dementia. Recent studies suggest that the prevalence of mixed dementia is greater than previously appreciated. Mixed dementia occurrence may also become more common with increasing age, because many of the dementias have similar risk factors.

- **Dementia with Lewy bodies (DLB)**: The pattern of cognitive decline in DLB can be similar to that in AD, involving memory impairment, poor judgment, and confusion. However, the individual may present with apathy more prominently in DLB than in Alzheimer's. The severity of cognitive symptoms and level of alertness may fluctuate from day to day. Individuals with DLB may experience excessive daytime sleepiness. Other common symptoms include visual hallucinations and Parkinsonian symptoms, such as "mask-like" face, rigidity, stiffness, shuffling gait, and problems with balance. About 50% of people with DLB experience rapid eye movement (REM) sleep behavior disorder (acting dreams out while sleeping, often having vivid dreams and acting out violently).

- **Parkinson's disease**: Parkinson's disease is classified primarily as a movement disorder, with symptoms including tremors and shakiness, stiffness, difficulty with walking and muscle control, lack of facial expression, and impaired speech. Many individuals with Parkinson's develop dementia in later stages of the disease. The medications used to treat Parkinson's disease can contribute to hallucinations and worsening of dementia.

- **Frontotemporal dementia (FTD)**: FTD represents a group of rare disorders in which neurodegeneration occurs. No single underlying pathological process is known. There are two types of FTD: Type 1 is defined by behavioral and personality changes that may include difficulty following social rules/norms and uncharacteristic impulsiveness and lack of inhibition; rudeness or tactlessness; poor financial judgment; inappropriate social conduct, sometimes extending into illegal activities; declining interest in grooming and hygiene; and overeating and weight gain. Individuals typically lack insight into such changes. This group of FTDs includes the well-known Pick's disease.

47

Type 2 is characterized by progressive disruption in verbal and written expression (primary progressive aphasia) or naming and understanding meaning (semantic dementia). Memory and other cognitive functions remain relatively unaffected. It tends to impact younger individuals, usually beginning between the ages of 35 and 75. Due to its earlier onset and prominent behavioral and personality symptoms, it may be mistaken for a primary psychiatric disorder. Most individuals with FTD perform poorly on neuropsychiatric tests of executive function. Brain imaging may show damage to the anterior temporal and frontal lobes.

- **Creutzfeldt-Jakob disease (CJD)**: CJD is a rare degenerative disorder affecting about 1 in 1,000,000 people worldwide annually. Most cases are sporadic and appear in individuals older than 60 years. About 5 to 10% of U.S. cases are inherited. Occasionally, it is infectious, as a result of exposure to contaminated medical instruments or transplant of infected tissues. It is a fast-progressing disorder and may initially involve impairment of just one of the major cognitive domains. It may also involve depression, anxiety, agitation, or changes in personality or behavior. Motor difficulties may occur from the beginning of symptom initiation or may appear shortly after cognitive and behavioral symptoms. These include involuntary muscle jerks and akinetic mutism (the person seems to be alert and can follow things with his or her eye movements but has no speech or voluntary movements). World Health Organization diagnostic criteria include at least one of the following laboratory findings: (1) an electroencephalogram typical for CJD or (2) presence of 14-3-3 protein in cerebrospinal fluid. Variant CJD is a related disorder recently identified in the United Kingdom. It has been linked to the consumption of beef or other products from cattle infected with bovine spongiform encephalopathy, or "mad cow disease."

- **Normal pressure hydrocephalus (NPH)**: NPH is a rare disorder that involves the build-up of fluid in the brain. It typically has three symptoms: difficulty walking, loss of bladder control, and mental decline. The person may respond slower, with cognitive functions becoming delayed, but the individual tends to be accurate and appropriate to a situation. Gait problems and incontinence are common in the late stages of all dementias, but they are rarely prominent early features except in NPH.

- **Huntington's disease**: This is a fatal genetic brain disorder. It has a strong genetic link: For those with a parent with Huntington's disease, there is a 50% chance of inheriting the disease. In 1 to 3% of cases, no history of the disease can be found in other family members. The age when symptoms develop and rate of progression vary from person to person. Symptoms include involuntary movements such as twitches and muscle spasms; problems with balance and coordination; personality changes, such as irritability, depression, and mood swings; and trouble with memory, concentration, and making decisions.

- **Korsakoff syndrome**: This brain disorder appears to have a link to vitamin deficiency: It is characterized by a lack of thiamine (vitamin B1). It involves two separate phases: *Wernicke encephalopathy* is the first, acute phase, and *Korsakoff psychosis* is the long-lasting, chronic stage. Symptoms of Wernicke-Korsakoff syndrome include
  - » Confusion, permanent gaps in memory, and difficulty learning new information.
  - » A tendency to confabulate, or make up, information and stories when the person has trouble remembering. The individual is not necessarily lying: He or she may actually believe the invented explanation.
  - » Unsteadiness, muscle weakness, and lack of coordination.

  The most common risk factor is alcoholism, but the syndrome can also be associated with other disorders, such as AIDS, cancers that have spread through the body, very high levels of thyroid hormone, and other conditions. Recent research suggests that APOE e4, a variant of a gene that produces the protein apolipoprotein E, may be associated with a higher risk of Wernicke-Korsakoff in individuals who drink heavily.

Treatment for Alzheimer's Disease
Cholinesterase inhibitors and N-methyl-D-aspartate Receptor Antagonists

Treatment of AD is currently aimed at slowing the disease progression, improving quality of life, and managing the problems that result as the disease progresses. As mentioned previously, there are several types of medications used to treat the associated memory loss, behavior changes, sleep problems, and the other symptoms of AD. It should be noted that all medications used in management of AD, as well as any of the other dementias, can have side effects, which can be even more pronounced in elders.

There are two classes of drugs that have been approved by the FDA for treating AD (Table 3-3): cholinesterase inhibitors and N-methyl-D-aspartate (NMDA) receptor antagonist. The first class of drugs discussed is the cholinesterase inhibitors. In the brains of individuals with AD, acetylcholine is destroyed too rapidly, making it difficult for the signals to be transmitted along the neural pathway. Cholinesterase inhibitors are used to slow the destruction of acetylcholine and thus slow the progression of AD and help improve cognition and cognitive symptoms. Cholinesterase inhibitors work by preventing the breakdown of acetylcholine, which is important for learning, memory, and attention. There are three cholinesterase inhibitors approved for the treatment of AD, which are indicated and approved to treat mild, moderate, and severe AD: donepezil (Aricept), rivastigmine (Exelon), and galantamine (Razadyne). Rivastigmine (Exelon) is also approved to treat Parkinson's disease dementia. Common side effects for any of these cholinesterase inhibitors include nausea, vomiting, diarrhea, weight loss, and dizziness. Another side effect of cholinesterase inhibitors includes symptomatic bradycardia and syncope, which may lead to falls (Thompson et al., 2004).

The second class of drugs approved by the FDA to treat AD is NMDA receptor antagonists. There is only one medication in this class: memantine (Namenda). This drug works by regulating the amount of another chemical messenger in the brain called glutamate, which is made in excess in the moderate and late stages of AD. Excessive glutamate interferes with information retrieval and memory and causes behavioral problems and impulsiveness. Namenda is indicated and approved by the FDA for treating the moderate to severe stages of AD and works by binding with the excessive glutamate. Side effects can include dizziness, confusion, headache, constipation, nausea, and agitation. Because Namenda works on a different chemical within the brain than a cholinesterase inhibitor, the two types of drugs are often used in combination.

[see **Table 3-3.** on page 52]

Table 3-3. Medications Indicated and Approved to Treat Alzheimer's Disease

Medication Class	Benefits	Medication and Dosage
Cholinesterase inhibitors	Slows the destruction of acetylcholine May improve cognition: Possibly improves MMSE score by 1 point (average untreated person sees MMSE score drop by 2–4 points annually) Cognitive benefits are sustained over 1–2 yr	Donepezil (Aricept) • 5 mg daily for 1 months, then 10 mg daily • New 23-mg dose available as daily dose if appropriate in patient who has been on 10 mg daily for at least 3 months Ravistigmine (Exelon) • Start at 1.5 bid, increase every 2 weeks to 3 mg bid, then 4.5 mg bid, then 6 mg bid (optimal/max. dose, 12 mg daily) • Available as patch, 4.6 mg/24 hr, applied daily for 2 weeks, then 9.5 mg/24 hr applied daily • New 13.3-mg/24 hr patch available for use after patient has been on 9.5-mg patch for 3 months Galantamine (Razadyne) • 4mg bid; increase every 4 weeks (max dose, 12 mg bid)
NMDA receptor antagonists	Regulates the production of glutamate and binds with excess glutamate Calms agitation and other behavioral problems May slightly improve memory retrieval	Memantine HCL (Namenda) • Start at 5 mg daily for 1 week, increase to 5 mg bid for 1 week, then 5 mg in morning and 10 mg in evening for 1 week, then 10 mg bid • May stop at 5 mg bid for patients who have renal impairment

bid = twice a day

Other Medications: Antidepressants

Antidepressants are widely used in individuals with AD because of the high rate of depression seen in individuals with Alzheimer's disease (30–50%; Aboukhatwa et al., 2010). Depression can be a risk factor for the development of AD or can be developed secondary to the neurodegenerative process. Some studies have shown that antidepressants may reduce the ominous brain plaques associated with AD (Sanders, 2011). Although there are several classes of antidepressants, the SSRI class is the most commonly used type of antidepressant in the older population, especially those with AD, because of their therapeutic efficacy and favorable side-effect profile (Brown et al., 2009). SSRIs selectively inhibit the reuptake of serotonin and subsequently increase the amount of serotonin available to bind to the postsynaptic receptor (Aboukhatwa, 2010). They are highly selective in treating depression symptoms and are well known for their benign interaction. SSRIs have been shown to be just as effective as an antipsychotic for calming agitation and treating psychotic symptoms in older individuals with dementia and may offer them a far safer alternative to conventional treatment with antipsychotic medications (Chow et al., 2007).

[see **Table 3-4.** on page 54]

Table 3-4. Selective Serotonin Reuptake Inhibitors*	
Drug	**Dosage**
Bupropion (Wellbutrin)	75–100 mg qd or bid
Duloxetine (Cymbalta)	20–60 mg qd
Escitalopram (Lexapro)	5–20 mg qd
Fluoxetine (Prozac)	10–20 mg qd
Paroxetine(Paxil)	10–40 mg qd
Paroxetine CR (Paxil CR)	12.5–37.5 mg qd
Sertraline (Zoloft)	25–50 mg qd
Venlafaxine XR (Effexor XR)	37.5–150 mg qd
*Approved by the FDA to treat depression. Side effects include weight gain, dizziness, somnolence, insomnia, decreased libido and other sexual side effects, tremors, akathesia, tremors, nervousness, sweating, and various gastrointestinal side effects.	
bid = twice a day; qd = once a day	

Other Medications: Anxiolytics, Antipsychotics, and Anticonvulsants

Antipsychotic medications and hypnotic/anxiolytic drugs are commonly prescribed to people with AD for the behavior or mood disturbances that commonly occur with the disease. A study demonstrated that their use was associated with an increased risk of mental deterioration. The older generation of antipsychotic drugs (haloperidol) tended to associate stronger with the rate of progression than atypical antipsychotic drugs (Ellul et al., 2007).

Anxiety is common problem in individuals with dementia. Anxiolytics are a class of anti-anxiety medications used to treat anxiety. They work by calming and relaxing a person. Anxiolytics are helpful when a confused individual is unable to be consoled, redirected, or calmed and may injure self or others. These medications do have side effects, including sleepiness, fainting, dizziness, blurred vision, confusion, and potential falls due to their effects on balance. There are risks if prescribed in high doses. Anxiolytics can potentially interact with alcohol or other drugs, causing depression of brain functioning, which can cause respiratory depression and even death. Anxiolytics should be used cautiously but may be necessary when an individual is unable to function and has a poor quality of life due to anxiety, paranoia, or extreme delusions.

Antipsychotic medications are another class of medications that have historically been used to calm the behaviors in individuals with AD, although they are not indicated for treatment of the disease. They have been used in individuals with dementia to treat the psychotic symptoms, such as hallucinations, delusions, or extreme "sundowning" behaviors (increased confusion and restlessness in the evening in people with dementia). Antipsychotic medications are also used to decrease racing thoughts, paranoia, and agitation and can allow a person to interact with others in a calmer manner, follow a routine, and be as independent as possible. However, antipsychotic medications can also cause mental slowing and lead to falls and other complications.

The benefits of using this type of medication must be weighed against the risks. This class of drugs must not be used as a chemical restraint (i.e., when a medication is used to subdue a person through sedation). It is important to note that older individuals may have problems when taking an antipsychotic medication. The adverse effects may include an increased risk of strokes and death, worsening of diabetes, worsening of cholesterol problems, and increased risk of injury related to falling. These drugs currently have a "black box" warning issued by the FDA about their use in the elderly with dementia for increased risk of death. Antipsychotic medications can also cause dystonia — abnormal, repetitious, involuntary movements, such as constant tongue protrusion, constant chewing, rocking motions, and pill rolling. If an individual develops dystonic movements, medication use must be re-evaluated to determine if continued use is in the person's best interest or if the medication should be discontinued. Appropriate laboratory monitoring is required with the use of all of the antipsychotic medications, including tests to monitor liver and kidney functioning, tests of glucose and hemoglobin A1c to monitor status of diabetes, and cholesterol panels at least every 6 months.

Additional medications are used in the management of the symptoms of AD and other dementias. Anticonvulsants have been used to manage behavioral problems in certain psychiatric illnesses, as well as dementia. The most commonly used drug in this class is valproic acid (Depakote), which has been used to treat epilepsy, bipolar disorder, and migraine headaches. Psychiatrists observed that valproic acid had certain side effects including calming of anxious behaviors. It then began to be used for these effects on mood and behavior in individuals with behavioral problems.

Valproic acid dampens the speed and frequency with which neurons fire. In addition to assisting in managing anxiety, agitation, and psychotic behaviors in individuals with dementia, scientists also think that valproic acid may inhibit the development of the plaques and tangles in the brains of people with AD (Peterson, 2004). This medication should be used cautiously because it has the potential to cause sedation, falls, and orthostatic hypotension (blood pressure dropping, which can lead to lightheadedness and falls). There is a "black box" warning for liver damage, and people taking this medication must undergo routine monitoring of liver function and drug levels to monitor for and prevent toxicity. Be aware that for dementia, the level of valproic acid in an individual's blood does not need to be in the therapeutic range, since it is not being used to treat seizures.

[see **Table 3-5.** on page 57]

Table 3-5. Antipsychotic and Anticonvulsant Medications Used With Dementia

Medication Class	Medication	Dosage
Anti-psychotics*	Aripiprazole (Abilify)	2–30 mg qd or bid
	Haloperidol (Haldol)	0.5–5 mg bid or tid
	Olanzapine (Zyprexa)	1.25–10 mg qd at bedtime or bid
	Quetiapine (Seroquel)	12.5–200 mg qd, bid or tid
	Risperidone (Risperdal)	0.25–1 mg qd or bid
	Ziprasidone (Geodon)	20–80 mg qd or bid
Anti-convulsants†	Valproic acid (Depakote)	125–500 mg qd or bid

*Not indicated by the FDA for treating behavioral problems in elders with dementia. Indicated for use with agitation and psychosis in individuals with psychosis, bipolar disorder, and other psychiatric conditions. All patients receiving drugs in this class must have routine monitoring of liver and kidney functioning, hemoglobin A1c, and cholesterol. Side effects include hypotension, hypertension, seizures, hyperglycemia, worsening of diabetes, weight gain, headache, cataract formation, worsening of depression, and hyperprolactinemia. Antipsychotics also have the potential to cause sedation, somnolence or insomnia, orthostatic hypotension, falls, strokes, diabetes, extrapyramidal symptoms, dystonic movements, myocardial infarction, QT prolongation, and death.
†Indicated by the FDA for treatment of seizure disorder. Not indicated by the FDA for use of managing behavioral problems in elders with dementia. Side effects include somnolence, dizziness, falls, orthostatic hypotension, increased confusion, and liver toxicity. All patients receiving this medication must have routine monitoring of liver functioning and valproic acid levels.
qd = once a day; bid = twice a day; tid = three times a day.

Lifestyle With Alzheimer's Disease

Individuals who have AD seem calmer and experience less agitation/acting out behaviors when they have a regular daily routine. Often people with AD need help handling routine daily activities, such as bathing, dressing, eating, and using the bathroom. If the caregiver can establish a daily schedule, it will assist in making the day go smoother. Although the schedule must be flexible to allow for the person to make some decisions about his or her routine and life, a daily routine helps give the individual some familiarity and control of his or her environment. The following factors are important in creating a routine. Managing AD symptoms through lifestyle factors is discussed in greater detail in Chapters 6 and 7.

- Routine, routine, routine
- Controlling environmental factors (e.g., decreasing noise and activity in the person's environment)
- Memory therapy (e.g., read old books, watch old movies, reminisce)
- Exercise (non-demanding, non-stressful repetitive exercises)
- Activities
  » Meeting the person's abilities
  » Not requiring the learning of new information
  » Non-demanding expectations
- Anti-stress measures (e.g., walking, listening to music, reading a book to the person)
- Music therapy with music of the person's preference

Communication in Alzheimer's Disease

The following principles for communicating with individuals suffering from dementia may diminish the incidence of certain behavioral problems that can arise. Good communication can create an environment that is less stressful and will likely improve the quality of life for both the person with AD and those caring for him or her. These suggestions also enhance the caregiver's ability to handle day-to-day life (Caregiver.org, 2010).

1. **Set a positive mood for interaction.** Pay careful attention to mannerisms, attitude, and body language — the individual's as well as the caregiver's. Set a positive mood by speaking in a pleasant and respectful manner. Use facial expressions, an even tone of voice, and physical touch to help maintain a humanistic relationship with the person as well as convey messages. When an individual is agitated and behaving aggressively, speak to the person in an even, monotone voice with a matter-of-fact tone and do not tense up with aggressive or defensive body language. (Agitated individuals usually react to the response they receive; e.g., if the caregiver responds as with surprise and an upset manner, the person may become more defensive and upset, further escalating the problem.)

2. **Get the person's attention.** Limit distractions and noise — it may be helpful to eliminate background noise by turning off the radio or television, close the curtains, shut the door, or consider moving to a quieter area when trying to communicate or accomplish a task with the person. Address the person by name, identify yourself by name and relation, and use nonverbal cues, such as hand signals or attempt to demonstrate the action the caregiver wishes the person to emulate. Consider using touch to keep the person engaged and focused. Speak at the person's educational level, maintain eye contact, and if possible, do not stand in a dominating position, as this may make the person feel threatened (e.g., when the person is seated, don't stand to the side and look down at him or her).

3. **Use simple words, concrete terms, and short single sentences but not "baby" talk.** Attention should be given to using terminology that is simple and concrete. Sentences should be short and concise so the person

can follow the train of thought or instruction. When a discussion or explanation is lengthy or a long series of instructions is given, the person may become lost and forget the first things said, due to memory impairment. Abstract words may not be understood or may be confused with a concrete definition. For example, do not say "hop on the bed," as the person may not understand that the caregiver wants him or her to sit on the bed; it would be more appropriate to simply say "please sit on the bed."

4. **Make speech heard clearly.** Speak slowly, distinctly, and in a reassuring tone; refrain from using a high or overly loud tone of voice. Instead, attempt to lower the pitch of your voice, as some older individuals who have some degree of hearing loss hear lower tones more clearly than higher ones.

5. **Ask simple, answerable questions.** Ask one question at a time and refrain from asking open-ended questions, such as "What would you like to eat?" Also, do not give a person too many choices or he or she may be overwhelmed and not able to make a decision. It is better to ask questions that offer limited choices, such as "Would you like to eat a hamburger or a salad?" Make an effort not to ask questions that can be answered with yes or no response, such as "Do you need to use the bathroom?" Instead, ask leading questions/statements, such as "Let's go try to use the bathroom, okay?"

6. **Break down activities into a series of steps.** Offer one instruction at a time, and allow the person to complete the requested task before offering another instruction. This makes many tasks more manageable. Encourage the person to do what he or she is able to, gently remind him or her of steps that were forgotten, and assist with steps he or she is no longer able to accomplish without assistance. Use visual cues, such as pointing to where the

person should sit, demonstrating how to put toothpaste on a toothbrush.

7. **When the going gets tough, distract and redirect.** When a person becomes upset, attempt to redirect his or her attention away from the cause of anger to help him or her calm down. Try talking about something else or changing the subject or the environment, such as talking about the weather or what the person is wearing. You can also encourage the person to do another task; for example, "Let's go see what you would like to wear tomorrow" or "I wonder where Edna is. Let's go see if we can find her."

Environment

Keeping the environment simple, uncluttered, and easy to maneuver through and having made as few changes as possible from how it was before the person developed symptoms have been shown to diminish behavioral problems in individuals suffering from dementia. A person's environment is the key to making his or her world as stress free as possible.

Modifying Environment

Caregivers who must manage problematic behaviors in confused individuals must be creative in developing strategies to prevent and diminish problems and calm an agitated individual. Structuring the environment is essential, and being knowledgeable of an array of maneuvers when one technique does not work will assist in decreasing the occurrence of problematic behaviors and mitigating problems when they do occur. Many times, the approaches a caregiver takes in creating a safe and effective environment can either make the situation better or cause it to become worse. See the following table for some ideas.

[see **Table 3-6** on page 62]

Table 3-6. Suggestions for Creating a Safe and Effective Environment for a Person With Dementia

Color and Pattern

- To draw the person's attention to something, use bright and/or eye-catching colors, such as stark white, yellow, orange, red, and black.
- For a calming effect, use soothing colors, such as peach, pink, beige, ivory, light blues, greens, and lavender.

- To assist in the person's ability to see objects more clearly (e.g., countertops, doorway to the bathroom, food), use high-contrast colors, such as red doorways with pastel walls, red plates on white tablecloths, or brightly colored plates with light-colored food.
- To mask or "hide" things (such as doors the person should not use), use similar colors (e.g., make the color of the door and door handle the same as the wall).
- Avoid the use of busy patterns on things such as in furniture, wallpaper, and flooring, which can appear as movement to a person with depth perception issues and can have a negative impact on a person's balance and cause falls: This problem is common in individuals with dementia.
- Avoid shiny flooring or windows, which may cause glare and prevent the person from seeing obstacles in his or her path. Consider use of diffuse lighting and covering windows with blinds, shades, or drapes.

Simplicity

- Maintain a clutter-free environment, because too many distractions or trinkets can be confusing and upsetting for individuals with dementia.
- Clear the walking paths of furniture, which can cause falls, especially the paths to the bathroom and kitchen.

Table 3-6. Safety (continued)

Orientation to Environment
- Use labels, pictures, and numbers to help the individual know where he or she is or what an object is.
- Leave notes to remind the person of things he or she needs to do, such as brush teeth, eat lunch, or change clothes.

Safety
- Use safety measures to prevent falls.
  » Area rugs or throw rugs can move when stepped on and cause falls — use double-sided tape on the backs.
- Remove harmful objects the person cannot use safely (e.g., knives, razors, power tools, guns).
- Be aware of plants that can be toxic if ingested.
- Place medications out of reach to prevent overdosing.
- Place twist-bolt or childproof locks on exterior doors to prevent the person from wandering off. Place locks high or low enough so that the person is unable to reach them easily.
- If using deadbolt locks, keep an extra set of keys near the door for easy accessibility but out of sight, so the person will not use them.
- Remove locks from bathrooms or bedrooms so the individual cannot get locked inside.
- Childproof locks or doorknobs can assist in limiting access to areas that contain harmful objects, such as knives, dangerous tools, cleaning supplies, or poisonous products.
- Child gates can prevent a confused person from falling down stairs or entering rooms that are off limits.
  » Wearing socks increases a person's risk for slipping and falling — use socks or slippers with grippers on the bottom.
  » Poor-fitting shoes can cause falls.
  » Pets can get under the person's feet and cause falls.

Table 3-6. Safety (continued)

- Decrease auditory stimulation.
  » Use carpet, which absorbs noise and prevents falls.
  » Limit distractions and control noise levels.
- Decrease visual stimulation, which can causes hallucination or delusions.
  » Avoid lighting that casts shadows to diminish hallucinations.
  » Use natural light and focus it directly on the areas where needed as much as possible.
- Use non-absorbent material to cover furniture in case of accidents or spills or buy furniture that is easy to wipe down but comfortable (such as a leather or vinyl recliner).
- Limit the use of certain appliances in the bathroom, such as electric razors or hairdryers, to reduce the risk of electrical shock.

Creativity
- Use memory aids, such as reminder notes, calendars, labels, or photographs. You may wish to display older photographs that match the era in which the person's clearest memories lie.
- Place large black rugs in front of doorways through which you do not wish a person to go: Individuals with dementia have a problem with depth perception, making rugs appears as holes, so many will avoid walking over a dark rug.
- Make the doorknob the same color as the door or cover the door with a picture, so it blends into the wall.
- When you wish the person to use a particular door, such as that for the bathroom, paint the doorframe a bright color that is different than the door.
- If a person frequently hides an object and then thinks someone has stolen it, is always looking for a certain thing, or wants to wear the same shirt every day, have multiples of the item to give the person when he or she becomes obsessed over it.

Planning

Planning for the future is essential for individuals with AD, such as decisions about stopping driving, moving the person out of his or her home into either a relative's house or a nursing home and, eventually, end-of-life decisions, such as feeding tubes. Staying in the home environment is optimal for most people to maintain routine and a sense of normalcy. It is often encouraged to maintain a person in his or her usual living environment for as long as possible. However, safety and the person's well-being are major considerations that may necessitate a change and require placement in a more structured environment. Such decisions depend on many factors, including:

- Severity of the individual's dementia
- How disruptive the person's behavior is
- Home environment and safety factors
- Availability of family members and caregivers
- Financial resources
- Presence of other unrelated disorders and physical problems

Strategies for Managing Disruptive Behaviors
Redirection

Redirecting and diverting an individual's attention away from whatever he or she is upset or stressed about to something that is more pleasant can be helpful. For example, when a person insists, "I need to get to the kids from school," you might say, "Okay, but how about we see what's for dinner first, since we have a few more minutes until the kids are out of school." Obviously, this technique's usefulness depends on what seems sensible in a given situation. Be creative and experiment to see what works and what doesn't. When redirection does not seem to be working, try asking pointed questions to get to the bottom of any unexplained behavior. Do not attempt to make the person explain his or her behavior; instead, attempt to discover the motivation for the behavior. This will make it easier to redirect if you understand what the person is thinking or why he or she is upset (Gilbert Guide, n.d.).

Validation Therapy

Validation therapy, first conceived by Naomi Feil, combines bluntly explaining reality with allowing individuals suffering from dementia to believe what they want to believe. It integrates redirection techniques (moving the person's attention from one thing to another) with validating and understanding the person's feelings and emotions. It is based on the idea that a person suffering from dementia may be sorting through past memories and past issues but living them out in the present. Some may even retreat to the past significantly to restore a feeling of balance and control, especially if their present memory is failing. Allowing these individuals to live in the past allows them some measure of control, which will aid in self-worth and reduce the occurrence of negative behaviors (Gilbert Guide, n.d.).

Try to understand why the person is behaving a certain way (e.g., what is the trigger or underlying concern?). Then attempt to figure out how to address the issue. For example, if the person is hoarding or hiding items, ask what he or she is fearful of losing. Give the person a "safe box" that can be used to store items about which he or she is obsessed. Do not attempt to make sense of a behavior — just accept the behavior and the person. An individual with dementia may seem lost or unable to complete a task and become frustrated. Remember that his or her emotions are still valid, and attempt to diminish frustrations by acknowledging them. In fact, a distressing or anxious behavior can be amplified when the person is not accepted or not understood. Accept that his or her emotions have more validity than the logic that leads the person to become frustrated. Ask specific questions about how certain actions or situations make him or her feel. After receiving an explanation of those feelings, validate the feelings with phrases that show acceptance and support, such as "I'd be upset, too, if that happened to me" or "I understand why you feel that way." Instead of arguing, allow the person a graceful exit from the conversation and be mindful of his or her ego (Gilbert's Guide, n.d.).

Structure and Stimulation

As stated earlier, individuals suffering from dementia usually function better in familiar surroundings and with an established routine. Problematic behaviors occur less often when he or she is within a structured and safe environment. Although the person's environment should be stable, it should also include some stimulation, such as an exercise program and verbal or auditory stimulation from conversations, radio, or television. The environment should help orient the person. For example, place the person near a window so he or she can differentiate day and night or put up decorations to remind the individual of holidays.

Structure and routine will assist in orienting a confused person and give him or her a sense of stability and security. When there are changes in routines, environment, or caregivers, simple and direct explanations should be given. Before every interaction, such as a bath or a meal, a confused person should be told what is going to happen. Taking time to explain can help prevent aggressive or combative behaviors. Following a daily routine for tasks can help the person with dementia remember to some degree. Establish a routine for bathing, eating, and sleeping (Merck, 2013a).

Activities should be scheduled on a regular basis to help people suffering from dementia have a better quality of life and feel independent, needed, and less depressed. Activities can be related to the individual's interests prior to dementia, should be enjoyable, and should provide stimulation but not be too challenging, which can cause frustration and aggression. Physical activity can relieve stress, expend a person's energy, and help prevent sleep problems as well as disruptive behaviors.

Staying active also helps improve balance, which may help prevent falls and maintain (or improve) overall health (Merck, 2013a).

Engaging a person suffering from dementia in activities will assist in keeping him or her more alert and possibly lead to a better disposition. For example, a person should be stimulated with mental activities such as hobbies, hearing about interesting current events, and being read to about past events, such as from old newspapers. Activities should not be demanding and may need to be broken down into small parts or simplified as dementia worsens. A person with dementia should not be isolated, but excessive stimulation should be avoided. Interaction with familiar people and socialization is encouraged. Activities should be incorporated into a simplified daily routine, expectations should be realistic, and structure should be predictable to maintain the person's dignity and self-esteem (Merck, 2013a).

CHAPTER 4

EARLY-ONSET
ALZHEIMER'S DISEASE

EARLY-ONSET AD AFFECTS YOUNGER ADULTS — SOMETIMES THOSE AS YOUNG AS 40 YEARS. THIS FORM OF AD USUALLY HAS A FASTER PROGRESSION THAN LATE-ONSET AD (WHICH TYPICALLY OCCURS AFTER THE AGE OF 65) AND OFTEN RUNS IN FAMILIES. THIS CHAPTER PRESENTS A DISCUSSION OF EARLY-ONSET AD AND HOW IT AFFECTS THE INDIVIDUAL AND FAMILY.

"You have forgotten one chapter in your latest book." This is the comment I received from a family member at one on my support group meetings. He told me that his wife has early-onset AD and it has been devastating for their preteen sons. Problems began when his wife was in her early 40s: She became lost in familiar places and irritable, with small lapses in memory. It is hard for the children to understand why Mom is not able to take care of them, to drive them to baseball practice, to help with homework, and just "be Mom." They are afraid that their friends (and other parents) will find out about her problems. It is even more difficult for this wonderful, caring man to watch his wife lash out at her children and no longer be the loving wife he once knew. This chapter is devoted to all families who are dealing with early-onset AD and the devastating consequences they must endure.

Nearly 5.2 million Americans are living with AD; although most are older than 65 years, approximately 5% have a form of the disease that develops in younger individuals — early-onset AD. This condition can be diagnosed in people in middle adulthood — in their 30s, 40s, and 50s (NINDS, 2014).

69

Early-onset AD is not as common as the late-onset form of the disease; it is often referred to as rare. Any individual who suspects that he or she or a family member has symptoms of AD should seek the advice of a health care provider immediately, regardless of age. There are ways to slow the progression of the disease through lifestyle measures and medications, including some promising new medications. Although the diagnosis is certainly scary, a proactive approach is not only practical but can give those affected some sense of control over what lies ahead (Alzheimer's Association, 2014j).

As mentioned in previous chapters, AD is generally characterized by the occurrence of a progressive dementia associated with cerebral cortical atrophy, beta-amyloid plaque formation, and intraneuronal neurofibrillary tangles. The presentation of the disease typically begins with subtle memory failure that progresses to more severe memory issues, behavioral problems, and eventual incapacitation. As noted, other associated symptoms include confusion, poor judgment, language disturbance, agitation, withdrawal, hallucinations, seizures, increased muscle tone, incontinence, and inability to speak (Bird, 2012). Familial AD (FAD), also referred to as early-onset AD, is characterized by AD running in families, with more than one member having it — usually multiple siblings in the same generation as well as other close relatives.

The term *familial* means that this variation of the disease is inherited, a genetic trait passed on through the genes from parents to children. Many individuals in the same family may be affected, since the disease is passed on through an autosomal, dominant gene (meaning a person can receive the gene from only one parent and develop the disease; Bird, 2012). There are three clinically indistinguishable subtypes of EOFAD based on the underlying genetic mechanism. These are: AD type 1 (AD1), caused by mutations in *APP* (10–15% of EOFAD); AD type 3 (AD3), caused by mutations in *PSEN1* (30–70% of EOFAD); and AD type 4 (AD4), caused by mutations in *PSEN2* (<5% of EOFAD). Other variations of this type of autosomal dominant EOFAD occur with no identifiable mutations in

PSEN1, PSEN2, or *APP*; thus, it is likely that there are other causes of these types of mutations (Bird, 2012). Molecular genetic testing for PSEN1, PSEN2, and APP is available and generally encouraged for brothers and sisters of an individual who has been diagnosed with EOFAD.

Warning Signs

There may be warning signs that there are problems in cognition, which may be a signal or early indicator of EOFAD. These signs are similar to those of late-onset AD and include regularly losing or misplacing items, having difficulty executing common tasks (e.g., cooking, writing checks, managing bills), forgetfulness, personality changes (e.g., depression, aggression, anxiety), confusion, poor judgment, having challenges with basic communication and language, social withdrawal, and problems following simple directions or a series of instructions.

Diagnosis

Early-onset AD or FAD is diagnosed in individuals with the following symptoms:

- Adult onset of a progressive dementia (before the age of 60 years)
- Absence of other causes of dementia
- Cerebral cortical atrophy, diagnosed by neuroimaging studies
- Beta-amyloid neuritic plaques and intraneuronal neurofibrillary tangles, diagnosed at autopsy if the person is deceased
- Family has more than one member with AD (usually multiple affected persons in more than one generation), and the age of onset is consistently younger than age 60 years, often before age 55 years

To establish the extent of disease in an individual diagnosed with EOFAD, perform the following as part of the diagnostic process:

- History
  - » Age of first symptom presentation (in particular, onset before age 45 years may indicate more rapid progression)
  - » Duration and progression of symptoms
- Examination (including laboratory and imaging studies)
  - » Physical examination (include laboratory work-up to rule out other causes)
  - » Cognition/mental status
  - » MRI, PET scan (severe cortical atrophy on MRI or marked metabolic deficits on PET imaging suggest more advanced disease)

Management

Early-onset AD can be difficult to cope with. The best plan of action is to have a positive outlook and stay as active and mentally engaged as possible. It's also important to realize that no one has to be alone in this disease. A person diagnosed with EOFAD should be encouraged to rely on friends and family as much as possible. No one should be afraid to seek out a support group, as this can be a wonderful source of support, knowledge about the disease, and suggestions on ways to cope and manage disease symptoms.

In the early stages of EOFAD, it is critical to plan ahead and think about the future. This can include doing financial planning, working with employers on current and potential job responsibilities, clarifying health insurance coverage, and getting all important documents in order, should an individual's health take a turn for the worse.

Treatment suggestions are the same as those in Chapter 3, "Diagnosing and Treating Alzheimer's Disease," which discusses the late-onset version of AD. In EOFAD, the main focus of treatment is supportive, and each symptom is managed on an individual basis. In general, affected individuals eventually require a caregiver to assist with basic activities (i.e., bathing, grooming, eating, toileting, walking/transferring) and managing executive functioning (i.e., housekeeping, shopping, cooking, driving, managing medications and managing affairs).

Although the exact biochemical basis of AD is not well understood, it is known that deficiencies of brain cell conduction and neurotransmitter chemical imbalances are present. Medications are used to slow the progression of chemical imbalances. Agents that increase cholinergic activity, making acetylcholine available for the neurons, such as tacrine, a cholinesterase inhibitor, are approved for treatment and show modest but variable benefit. These medications are donepezil (Aricept), rivastigmine (Exelon), and galatamine (Reminyl); (Bird, 2012). Memantine, an NMDA receptor antagonist, which binds with the excessive glutamate in the brain, has also been approved for use in AD.

A daily routine should be established, and the environment should be familiar, unchanging, and uncluttered. Medical and behavioral management of mood and behavior should be addressed: It is important to manage depression, aggression, sleep disturbance, seizures, and hallucinations. Medications are often used for these purposes and include antidepressants, particularly the SSRIs, such as citalopram (Celexa), escitalopram (Lexapro), sarafem fluoxetine (Sarafem), paroxetine (Paxil), and sertraline (Zoloft).

Lifestyle factors are also important in managing the symptoms of EOFAD. Following are some suggestions. (See Chapters 6 and 7 for more detail.)

- Physical and occupational therapy can be helpful to manage problems with gait (walking ability) and activities of daily living (i.e., bathing, grooming, transferring, continence, eating).
- Regular aerobic exercise (30 minutes three to five times a week) can help with general health, mood, and mobility; raise heart rate with activities such as steady walking, swimming, or stationary bicycling to increase blood flow to the brain.

- A healthy diet is also important. The following are some components:
  - » Low cholesterol
  - » Antioxidants (see Chapter 6 for more regarding diet)
  - » Regular intake of protein
  - » Avoidance of foods high in sugar or preservatives
- Routine exercise of the brain through reading (or listening to someone read), puzzles, games, learning something new in the early stages (e.g., auditing a college class, learning to knit) can help slow the progression of cognitive problems.
- Monthly evaluations should be done to monitor for further deterioration of abilities and rate of progression of the disease and to identify and manage secondary complications.
- Sudden changes in environment or routine should be avoided, because this can cause emotional outbursts and aggressive behaviors. Also, the use of certain medications and oversedation should be avoided, because more complications could occur.

Rate of Progression

As stated previously, younger individuals who exhibit symptoms of AD have a faster progressing disease process, a fact that was confirmed by a study conducted by Musicco and colleagues (2009). Many individuals with EOFAD still have children at home, and this can complicate many issues, including how the children will manage as the parent begins to exhibit psychiatric manifestations of the disease. The affected person and his or her spouse or partner may also have elderly parents who need care. It can often be overwhelming to care for an elderly parent, but caring for a parent as well as a loved one with EOFAD and children all at the same time can be debilitating.

Individuals with AD may continue to care for themselves, live in their own homes, and function independently as long as possible. Many resources are available for the family and the caregivers — support that can be essential when dealing with EOFAD.

Impact on the Person with Early-Onset Familial Alzheimer's and on Family Members

Alzheimer's disease affects each individual differently. Each person who develops EOFAD will progress through the disease in a unique manner. Each will have good days and bad days. It's important to try to maximize the good days and not dwell on the bad days, but instead to develop strategies to cope as well as possible in particular situations. Awareness is the key to preparing to manage life with AD and the problems that may occur. The same is true for family members of the person with EOFAD. Following are suggestions for both the affected individual and his or her loved ones. (See Chapter 8, for more detailed suggestions.)

The Individual With Alzheimer's Disease

No individual with AD needs to deal with it alone (i.e., without family or close friends). People with EOFAD should consider joining a support group. Call the local chapter of the Alzheimer's Association for information on groups specifically for people with EOFD. Following are additional suggestions:

- Don't keep fears and feelings inside. Talk to family, friends, and health care providers with concerns or problems. Also consider seeking professional counseling.

- Take care of yourself. Get regular check-ups, and follow the health care provider's recommendations about diet, exercise, and taking medications.

- Don't tune out family and friends. Share experiences of living with AD. Stay as active as possible for as long as possible. Invite friends to attend educational programs about AD so they can better understand it.

Career. As the disease progresses, a person with EOFAD may find job-related tasks more difficult to perform. The affected individual should plan when and what to tell an employer about the disease and at what point he or she should no longer work. He or she should make adjustments if necessary to be able to continue to work as long as possible. This will help to maintain income and independence and boost self-esteem. Consider asking to be placed in a position that better matches current skills and capabilities or to reduce work hours. Investigate all possible options, including early retirement, as well as ways to access all benefits available through an employer.

Financial and Legal Matters. Plan ahead for financial needs, knowing that eventually you will have to leave your job and lose income. Meet with a financial counselor who can help investigate insurance, investments, and other financial options.

Talk with family and health care providers about available medical treatments are and what you wish regarding your plan of care in various circumstances, including in the event you become unable to communicate your wishes. Every individual should prepare an advance directive, a legal document that outlines wishes for future medical treatment. Organize all financial and legal documents, as well as other important information (e.g., insurance policies [including health insurance policies, long-term care policies, and life insurance], Social Security information, wills) in one place, and let family and/or children know where to find them.

Prepare computer information, including a list of important websites and login information (i.e., IDs and passwords). Contact the local Alzheimer's Association or access more information through their website.

Family and Friends

Communication. When you have a loved one with EOFD, it's important to talk openly with him or her, especially when it's a spouse or partner, about issues that are important, such as finances, household and child-rearing responsibilities, and sexual intimacy. Be aware that the person's ability to perform any of these tasks will change as cognition and abilities decline. Look toward future caregiving needs, and try to make plans and decisions together, ahead of time.

Talk openly with children about the disease, symptoms, and expected progression. Understand that EOFAD affects the entire family, including children. In addition to being concerned about the affected family member, children may have understandable fears about developing AD themselves. When appropriate, include children in making decisions that affect the whole family. Encourage them to become involved in a support group. Individuals with EOFAD should consider recording their thoughts, feelings, wisdom and memories, so they may pass them on to their children.

Genetic Testing and Counseling. Whether to get genetic testing is a personal decision that each family member of someone with EOFAD must consider. Testing is highly encouraged for all first-degree relatives of someone with AD (i.e., sisters, brothers, children), since the best plan of action would be to establish a diagnosis and obtain medical care as soon as possible to slow the disease down.

It is suggested that anyone considering genetic testing should pursue genetic counseling to assist in preparing for the potential results/outcomes — to examine the pros and cons, prepare for how to handle the potential consequences of knowing, and get help with planning for the future. Some things to consider are how a positive test may affect your eligibility for medical insurance, long-term care, disability and life insurance. If a person knows that he or she carries the genetic factors for developing EOFAD and is prepared, he or she may be able to take steps to make it easier for him — or herself and family members to cope with the effects of AD.

CHAPTER 5

OVERVIEW OF RESEARCH ON PREVENTION AND TREATMENT OF ALZHEIMER'S DISEASE AND OTHER FORMS OF DEMENTIA

RESEARCHERS ARE PROPOSING THAT THERE ARE MANY HEALTHY WAYS TO PREVENT MCI, AD, AND VASCULAR DEMENTIA. THIS CHAPTER DISCUSSES CURRENT RESEARCH SUGGESTING HEALTHY-BRAIN LIFESTYLE AND EXERCISE STRATEGIES.

Can AD be prevented? That is the billion-dollar question and one which, if answered correctly, could improve the health care of millions of people, save billions of dollars in health care costs, and potentially stand to make history. Current research indicates that there's little we can do to prevent AD and other types of dementia but hope for the best and wait for a cure. However, recent studies are suggesting that there are certain factors that can reduce an individual's risk of developing AD, such as eating right, exercising, staying mentally and socially active, and reducing stress. Through leading a brain-healthy lifestyle, the severity of the symptoms of AD can be diminished and the advancement of the disease can be slowed down, or even reversed (Smith et al., 2013). Strategies to prevent AD are aimed at factors an individual can manipulate or control. While some factors, such as genetic factors inherited from parents, cannot be controlled, many lifestyle factors are within a person's ability to change (Smith et al., 2013).

There are six pillars of a brain-healthy lifestyle (Smith et al., 2013):
1. Healthy diet
2. Regular physical exercise
3. Regular brain exercise, or mental stimulation
4. Quality sleep
5. Stress management
6. An active social life

A person must address each of these lifestyle factors and strengthen each of the six pillars in daily life; this will lead to a healthier and hardier brain. When individuals lead a brain-healthy lifestyle, the brain will stay working stronger ... longer. These lifestyle factors are discussed in detail in Chapters 6 and 7.

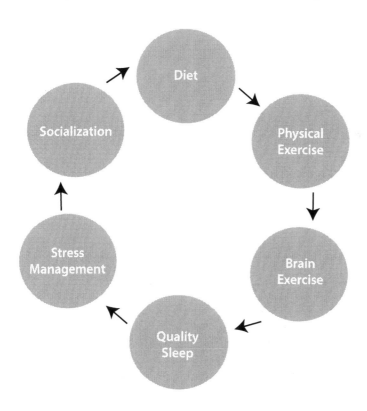

Genetics

The basic make-up of every human body begins with the genes each individual inherits from their parents, with each parent contributing half of their chromosomes. A basic explanation of human genetics begins with understanding the following (Merck, 2013b):

- A gene is a segment of DNA that contains the instructions used to synthesize a protein.

- A chromosome contains hundreds to thousands of genes.

- Every human cell contains 23 pairs of chromosomes (for a total of 46 chromosomes for each cell).

- A trait is a characteristic that a person develops based on an inherited gene or genes.

- Some traits are caused by abnormal genes that are inherited or that are the result of a mutation.

The Link Between Estrogen and Alzheimer's Treatment

As mentioned earlier, myloid plaques, one of the hallmark features of AD, form when clumps of beta-amyloid, a naturally occurring protein, build up between neurons in the brain, interfering with normal brain functioning. Research has suggested that estrogen may prevent the accumulation of beta-amyloid clumps in the brain, possibly by stimulating the breakdown of beta-amyloid proteins (MoreFocus, Alzheimers Disease Treatment, n.d.). This finding has increased researchers' interest in estrogen as a potential treatment for AD.

Hormone Therapy

Hormone therapy for AD has been investigated in the past, but no clear-cut evidence was found that it is effective; however, more research is being done in this arena. A recent study by Harvard and Stanford researchers proved that certain women who carry a well-known genetic risk factor for AD showed signs of more rapid aging in their body's cells than women who didn't have it. The researchers have indicated that this may be a link to understanding the role that the APOE e4 allele plays in the development of the disease. It has been estimated that 25 to 30% of the population carries at least one copy of APOE e4. Forty percent of people with AD do not exhibit the symptoms of the disease but can pass the gene on to their children (Konkel, 2013).

The study was conducted in a group of post-menopausal women whose average age was 58 years. These women were being voluntarily managed on hormone replacement therapy, either estrogen alone or estrogen plus progesterone, and were at risk for AD due to a family history of the condition. Of the 63 women in the study, only 24 were carriers of the APOE e4, the gene that predisposes an individual to developing AD. Half of these women were then randomly assigned to stop receiving hormone therapy, while half continued receiving it. After two years, the researchers found that the women who were APOE e4 carriers were six times more likely than non-carriers to exhibit obvious cellular aging once they stopped taking hormones. This suggests that, for women with this genetic variant (APOE e4 carriers), hormone replacement therapy may reduce the risk for cellular aging, which may also reduce their risk of dementia (Konkel, 2013).

The study had a limited number of participants, and it is unclear whether the protective effect the researchers saw was due to hormone replacement therapy or another factor. Recommendations on hormone therapy cannot be based on this study alone, and it remains unclear if hormone therapy will decrease risk of dementia. However, the results of this study do suggest that more investigation needs to be done to identify if and what type of hormone replacement therapy would be beneficial in preventing AD or as a treatment option for individuals with the disease (Konkel, 2013).

A larger study conducted by the Women's Health Initiative was begun in 1991 and ended in 2010. This study involved more than 160,000 generally healthy postmenopausal women and found that estrogen plus progestin therapy offered no protection against MCI in women older than 65 years. The women who took the hormones actually had an increased risk of dementia. The Women's Health Initiative is in the process of examining the effects of estrogen-only therapy on cognition (Konkel, 2013).

The Oxidation Theory

A leading theory is that free radical damage and oxidative stress cause aging and are also thought to play a major role in the development of AD. Oxidative stress can potentially damage an individual's DNA and affect cellular lipids, sugars, and proteins; any imbalance between the intracellular free radicals, reactive oxygen species, and antioxidant defense mechanisms results in oxidative stress (Aliev et al., 2008). It is thought that this is because neurons have an age-related decrease in the capacity to compensate for even minor cellular stresses, which may lead to irreversible injury.

A molecule carrying an unpaired electron (making it extremely reactive and ready to acquire an electron in any way possible from another molecule) is termed a *free radical*. However, as free radicals acquire an electron from other molecules, they either convert these molecules into other free radicals or break them down and alter their chemical structure. Thus, free radicals are capable of damaging virtually any biomolecule, including cellular proteins, sugars, fatty acids, and nucleic acids (Aliev et al., 2008). Free radical damage to long-lived biomolecules is a major contributor to cell death and can lead to cancer, heart disease, and other illnesses, including AD.

Exercise

According to the Alzheimer's Research & Prevention Foundation (2013), physical exercise reduces an individual's risk of developing AD by 50%. Regular exercise can also slow further deterioration in people who have begun to develop cognitive problems associated with AD. If a person has been inactive for a while, starting an exercise program can be intimidating. It can help to find small ways to add more movement into one's daily routine. Simple ways to increase activity include walking more by parking at the far end of the parking lot, taking the stairs, or walking around the block, doing laps in the living room, or pacing while talking on a cell phone.

Tips for getting started and sticking with an exercise plan include the following:

- **Exercise for at least 30 minutes three to five times per week.** Try walking, swimming, or any other activity that gets the heart rate up. Also consider adding routine household activities, such as gardening, cleaning, or doing laundry, which count as activity.

- **Build muscle to pump up the brain.** Moderate levels of weight and resistance training not only increase muscles; they also help maintain brain health. Combining aerobics and strength training is better than either activity alone. For those older than 65 years, adding two to three strength training sessions to the weekly routine may cut the risk of Alzheimer's in half.

- **Include balance and coordination exercises.** Head injuries from falls are an increasing risk as a person grows older, which in turn increases risk for AD and other forms of dementia. Balance and coordination exercises can help a person stay agile and avoid spills. Try yoga, Tai Chi, or exercises using balance discs or balance balls.

- **Stick with an exercise routine for at least a month.** It takes approximately 28 days for a new routine to become habit. A person should establish realistic goals on a workout calendar and post it where it can be seen daily. Build in a reward system. Quickly, the feel-good endorphins from regular exercise will help the person want to continue the exercise routine.

- **Protect the head.** Studies suggest that head trauma at any point in life significantly increases a person's risk of developing AD. This includes repeated hits in sports such as football, soccer, and boxing, or one-time injuries from a bicycle, skating, skateboarding, or motorcycle accident. Protect your brain by wearing properly fitting sports helmets, buckling seatbelts, and fall proofing the environment.

Controlling Hypertension

Hypertension is a condition in which the blood circulates through the arteries with too much force. People with hypertension are at elevated risk for heart disease and heart attacks, cerebrovascular disease and stroke, as well as aneurysms. Recently, there has been mounting evidence showing a correlation between cardiovascular health and brain health (Radiological Society of North America, 2007).

A study by Rodrigue and colleagues published in *JAMA Neurology* (2013) suggests that controlling or preventing hypertension earlier in life may limit or delay the brain changes associated with AD and other age-related neurological deterioration. The study looked at whether people with both hypertension and a common gene had more buildup of beta-amyloid proteins in the brain, a factor associated with the development of AD. Scientists believe amyloid is the first symptom of AD and that these plaques begin to develop a decade or more before symptoms of memory impairment and other cognitive difficulties begin. The APOE e4 allele is carried by 20% of the population.

Until recently, amyloid plaque could be seen only on autopsy, but new brain scanning techniques allow the plaque to be seen in living brains of adults who do not exhibit the symptoms of AD. Findings from both autopsy and amyloid brain scans show that at least 20% of typical older adults carry elevated levels of amyloid, a substance made up mostly of protein that is deposited in organs and tissues.

The conclusion drawn from this research is that controlling hypertension may significantly decrease a person's risk of developing amyloid deposits, even in those with genetic risk for AD. Rodrigue and colleagues (2013) noted that long-term studies are needed to verify that the use of hypertensive medications would consistently decrease amyloid deposits and thus decrease the likelihood of developing AD. Nevertheless, this early finding provides a window into the potential benefits of controlling hypertension that goes well beyond lowering the risk of heart disease, strokes, and other cardiovascular complications.

Scientists cannot fully explain the neural mechanisms underlying the effect of hypertension and APOE e4 on amyloid accumulation. However, earlier research has shown that chronic hypertension may enable easier penetration of the blood-brain barrier, resulting in more amyloid deposition. Conclusions have been made that controlling hypertension and maintaining good vascular health may limit or delay the brain changes associated with AD and other aging-related neurological deterioration.

Diabetes Mellitus

The increased incidence of diabetics developing AD is not completely understood. Diabetes leads to insulin resistance, which is a metabolic disorder characterized by diminished tissue sensitivity to insulin. Studies have shown that insulin resistance is associated with increased risk of cardiovascular disease, which has been linked with AD (Schwartz et al., 2013). Several studies indicate that people with diabetes, especially type 2, are at higher risk of eventually developing AD or other dementias. Taking steps to prevent diabetes, as well as promptly diagnose and control diabetes, may help reduce an individual's risk of developing AD.

Diabetes can cause several complications, including damage to the blood vessels, and is considered a risk factor for vascular dementia, which occurs due to brain damage that is often caused by reduced or blocked blood flow to the brain. Many people with diabetes have changes to the brain that are hallmark features of both AD and vascular dementia. Some researchers think that each condition fuels the damage caused by the other, and the two dementias may occur concurrently in an individual (Mayo Clinic, 2013).

The link between type 2 diabetes and Alzheimer's may occur as a result of how type 2 diabetes affects the ability of the brain and other body tissues to utilize sugar (glucose) and respond to insulin. Diabetes also may increase the risk of developing MCI. As noted previously, MCI is a condition in which people experience more cognitive problems and memory problems than are usually present in normal aging (Mayo Clinic, 2013).

Researchers continue to study the connections between diabetes and Alzheimer's and potential ways to prevent as well as treat diabetes and AD. For example, studies are examining medications used to treat type 2 diabetes to determine whether they also improve cognitive function in people with mild AD. Results are tentatively showing a positive change in cognitive function (Mayo Clinic, 2013). Taking steps to prevent or control diabetes may help reduce a person's risk of developing AD.

Hyperlipidemia/Dyslipidemia

Having elevated cholesterol levels, also referred to as hyperlipidemia or dyslipidemia, during middle age (age 30–50 years) predicts dementia later in life, and beta-amyloid deposition correlates with cholesterol levels among individuals with mild hyperlipidemia (Maki et al., 2005). Studies have shown that elevated total cholesterol levels, including an elevated low-density lipoprotein (LDL) level, are associated with increased cardiovascular disease and increased incidence of developing AD. Individuals can decrease the risk of hyperlipidemia and thus the risk of AD, by implementing a heart healthy diet, by establishing an exercise routine, and possibly by using medications to lower cholesterol levels. A class of medications called statins is commonly used to lower cholesterol levels, including LDL.

Sleep Problems

Research indicates that very short or long durations of sleep and inefficient sleep are associated with higher total cholesterol levels and increased risk of type 2 diabetes and hypertension (Schwartz et al., 2013). People who have poor sleep, including difficulty going to sleep, difficulty staying asleep at night, and early morning awakenings, may be at risk for developing AD risk factors (Exigence Group, 2012). A study investigating the correlation between poor sleep and AD showed that individuals who frequently wake up during the course of the night showed signs of amyloid plaque buildups in their brains. As previously noted, this is generally associated with the development of AD and is considered a major risk factor for developing the disease. Poor sleep has been shown to increase insulin resistance and incidence of diabetes mellitus type 2. Sleep problems can also lead to worsening of hypertension. As noted earlier in this book, both diabetes and hypertension are risk factors for developing AD.

Researchers have not been able to explain whether disturbed sleep causes the plaque buildups or if conditions that contribute to the development of AD, such as amyloid plaques, make it hard for a person to sleep. Nonetheless, establishing good sleeping habits is optimal.

Experts say there is no specific amount of sleep or "magic number" of hours a person needs each night. Different age groups need different amounts of sleep, and sleep needs are individual (National Sleep Foundation, 2013). That said, it has been suggested that sleeping seven to nine hours a night is ideal, and sleeping less than five hours a night is considered sleep deprivation and technically qualifies a person for a diagnosis of insomnia. If an individual experiences difficulty sleeping for a prolonged period, his or her health will begin to suffer, with worsening of diabetes and/or hypertension.

CHAPTER 6

DIETARY AND OTHER LIFESTYLE STRATEGIES FOR PREVENTING ALZHEIMER'S DISEASE

THIS CHAPTER DISCUSSES TECHNIQUES TO PREVENT AD, INCLUDING BRAIN-HEALTHY DIETARY PLANS AND THE TOP 10 BRAIN SUPER-FOODS, EXERCISE, AND OTHER LIFESTYLE STRATEGIES.

Myth or Truth: Exercise, diet, and brain games can prevent AD?

Although there are many stories from people saying they have prevented or reversed AD through controllable factors such as eating certain foods and avoiding others, increasing physical activity and exercising, and performing brain exercises, the scientific evidence is still unclear. However studies have found that eating a healthy diet, engaging in aerobic exercise on a regular basis, staying socially active, and keeping the mind engaged with games and puzzles are linked to lower odds of developing AD. Studies also suggest that these same lifestyle changes may also reduce the progression of symptoms for people who already have AD.

Seven dietary principles to reduce the risk of AD were presented at the International Conference on Nutrition and the Brain in Washington in July 2013:

1. Minimize intake of saturated fats and trans fats.

2. Include vegetables, legumes (beans, peas, and lentils), fruits, and whole grains as primary staples of the diet.

3. Eat one ounce of nuts or seeds (one small handful) daily (source of vitamin E).

4. Include vitamin B12 in your diet, fortified foods, or a supplement providing at least the recommended daily allowance (2.4 mcg per day for adults).

5. Choose a multiple vitamin without iron and copper.

6. Avoid the use of aluminum cookware, antacids, baking powder, or other products that contribute dietary aluminum.

7. Include aerobic exercise in a daily routine.

This chapter discusses these principles, as well as other dietary recommendations for preventing and slowing the progression of AD, as identified through research. Just like the rest of the body, the brain requires a nutritious diet to operate at its optimal level. For a healthy diet, many people focus on eating plenty of fresh fruit and vegetables, lean protein, and healthy fats. It has been suggested that eating foods to reduce inflammation and provide a steady supply of energy can arm the body and brain with the fuel to make the brain healthy and prevent, or at least slow, the processes of AD.

Diet
General Dietary Recommendations

For preventing or slowing AD, general guidelines include the following:

- **Minimize intake of saturated fats and trans fats.** See later in this chapter for more on this topic (Smith et al., 2013).

- **Eat four to six small, frequent meals** as opposed to one or two large meals a day. Eating in this style and at regular intervals helps the body to maintain consistent blood sugar levels. Avoid foods that increase blood sugar dramatically in a short period of time (such as refined carbohydrates high in sugar and white flour), which causes a rapid rise in blood glucose and may lead to inflammation of the brain (Smith et al., 2013).

- **Eat colorful foods.** Consider eating foods across the rainbow. Eat dark green leafy vegetables and colorful fruits, which span the color spectrum because they are rich in vitamins and antioxidants. Daily servings of berries and green leafy vegetables should be part of an individual's brain-protective routine. Vegetables, legumes (beans, peas, and lentils), fruits, and whole grains should be the primary staples of the diet (Smith et al., 2013).

- **Eat lots of antioxidants.** Antioxidants reduce inflammation and thus reduce the likelihood of developing AD. Substances with high antioxidant activity include anthocyanins, beta-carotene, catechins, coenzyme Q10, flavonoids (plant compounds that help with the body's circulation), lipoic acid, lutein, lycopene, selenium, and vitamins A, C, and E. Omega-3 fats, including fish oils (discussed separately), also have some antioxidant properties. See later in this chapter for more on antioxidants.

- **Eat lots of omega-3 fats.** Foods containing omega-3 fatty acids can help prevent AD and dementia, and researchers are actively pursuing this avenue in the search for a cure for AD. Food sources for omega-3 include cold-water fishes (e.g., salmon, tuna, trout, mackerel, and sardines). An alternative is taking a fish oil supplement (Smith et al., 2013).

  » Aim to eat at least two to three servings of oily fish each week to supply the body with inflammation-fighting compounds.

  » If you are concerned about environmental toxins, such as polychlorinated biphenyls (PCBs) in seafood, consider taking a high-purity fish oil supplement.

  » Alternative sources: Walnuts, flaxseeds, and dark green leafy vegetables are rich in the plant-based omega 3 precursor, alpha-linolenic acid (ALA).

- **Drink tea daily.** Regular consumption of green tea has been suggested to enhance memory and mental alertness and slow brain aging. White and oolong teas are also reported to be brain healthy. Drinking two to four cups of tea each day has proven benefits. Although not as powerful as tea, coffee also confers brain benefits when consumed in moderation (Smith et al., 2013).

- **Get enough vitamins.** The following vitamins have shown promise in preventing and/or slowing AD (see later in this chapter for more information):
  - » **Vitamin C:** Daily intake of this water-soluble vitamin can prevent colds and shorten the lifespan of a cold. It is an antioxidant that helps reduce the stress of oxidation — a phenomenon that is proposed to be a risk factor for AD. Vitamin C can be found in oranges, orange juice, yellow bell peppers, kiwi, strawberries, and other foods.
  - » **Vitamin E:** This fat-soluble vitamin can help protect against heart disease, cancer, and age-related eye damage (macular degeneration). It also helps with brain health. One ounce of nuts or seeds (one small handful), one cup of spinach, avocados, or shrimp provides a healthful source of vitamin E.
  - » **Vitamin B12:** A reliable source of vitamin B12, such as fortified foods or a supplement providing at least the recommended daily allowance (2.4 µg per day for adults) should be part of a daily diet. Clams pack a whopping 98.9 µg (1648% of the RDA) of vitamin B12 in just a 100-g serving. Alternative sources include oysters, mussels, fish, shrimps, scallops, liver of most animals, and beef. Lower levels of vitamin B12 can also be found in seaweeds, yeasts, and fermented foods like miso and tempeh.
  - » **Folate:** A person with folate deficiency is 3.5 times more likely to develop dementia. One cup of asparagus will fulfill nearly 66% of daily folate needs. Alternative sources include citrus fruits, beans (sprouting maximizes their nutrients and enhances absorption),

broccoli, cauliflower, beets, lentils, and leafy green vegetables, such as spinach and turnip greens.

» When selecting multiple vitamins, choose those without iron and copper, and consume iron supplements only when directed by a health care practitioner.

- **Modest red wine drinking** may have a protective effect on cognitive function and decrease the risk of AD and dementia due to the high levels of flavonoids and possibly other polyphenolics, such as resevratrol. However, wine-drinking is a double-edged sword, because excessive alcohol intake can lead to dementia and a host of other serious health conditions, such as cancer, by triggering chronic inflammation. Therefore, limit red wine to no more than one glass a day if you choose to drink.

- **Avoid aluminum.** Although aluminum's role in AD remains a matter of investigation, it is prudent to avoid the use of cookware, antacids, baking powder, or other products that contribute dietary aluminum.

Saturated and Trans Fats

A healthy diet that limits or eliminates foods high in saturated and trans fats can reduce the risk of heart problems and overweight and may also reduce the risk of AD. Saturated fat is found in dairy products (especially full-fat products, such as cream and butter), meats, and certain oils (coconut and palm); trans fats are found in many snack foods (such as pastries) and fried foods and are listed on labels as "partially hydrogenated oils."

Researchers with the Chicago Health and Aging Project followed participants in a study on the impact of saturated fat on AD over a four-year period. Those who consumed a diet high in saturated fat (around 25 g/day) were two to three times more likely to develop AD, compared with participants who consumed a diet lower in saturated fats (around 12 g/day or less) (Morris et al., 2003). Similar studies conducted in New York and Finland found results comparable to those of the Chicago study: People who consumed more "bad" fats were more likely to develop AD, compared with those who consumed less (Laitinen et al., 2006; Luchsinger et al., 2002). Not all researchers are in agreement. For example, a study in the Netherlands found no protective effect of avoiding "bad" fats (Engelhart et al., 2002).

The reason why certain fats may influence the brain remains poorly understood. Studies suggest that high-fat foods and increases in blood cholesterol concentrations may contribute to the production of beta-amyloid plaques in the brain, a hallmark of AD. These same foods increase the risk of obesity and type 2 diabetes, common risk factors for AD (Physician's Committee, 2013).

Vegetables, legumes (beans, peas, and lentils), fruits, and whole grains have little or no saturated fat or trans fats and are rich in vitamins that have protective properties for brain health, such as folate and vitamin B6. Diets that emphasize these foods are associated with low risk for weight problems and type 2 diabetes; they also appear to reduce risk for cognitive problems. The Chicago Health and Aging Project tracked study participants 65 years and older, and found that a high intake of fruits and vegetables was associated with a reduced their risk of cognitive decline (Morris et al., 2006). Specific healthy diets are discussed in more detail later in this chapter.

Cholesterol and APOE e4

High cholesterol levels have been linked to an increased risk for developing AD. A large study of Kaiser Permanente patients showed that participants with cholesterol levels greater than 250 mg/dL after the age of 40 had a 50% higher risk of AD three decades later, compared with participants with cholesterol levels below 200 mg/dL (Solomon et al., 2009). As noted previously, the APOE e4 allele, which is strongly linked to AD, produces a protein that plays a key role in cholesterol transport. It has been hypothesized that individuals with the

APOE e4 allele may absorb cholesterol more easily from their digestive tracts compared with people without this allele.

Vitamins

Vitamin E is an antioxidant found in many foods, particularly nuts and seeds, and is associated with reduced incidence of AD. Eating a small handful of typical nuts or seeds, which contain about 5 mg of vitamin E, is recommended daily. Other healthful food sources include mangoes, papayas, avocadoes, tomatoes, red bell peppers, spinach, and fortified breakfast cereals.

Vitamin D offers neuro-protective effects as well as anti-inflammatory effects on the brain. Vitamin D receptors and vitamin D–activating enzymes are abundant in the brain, and studies show that the brain uses high levels of vitamin D. One meta-analysis of the risk factors for AD showed that individuals with AD had lower serum vitamin D concentrations than those who did not develop AD (Annweiler et al., 2013). This reinforces the conceptualization of vitamin D as a "neurosteroid hormone" and a potential biomarker of AD. Vitamin D is a fat-soluble vitamin that can be found in fish, oysters, fortified cereals, and dairy products. Vitamin D blood levels should be 30 to 100 ng/mL. If a person has an extremely low level, he or she may be prescribed high doses of vitamin D (i.e., 50,000 IU daily or weekly) until the level is adequate. Normal recommended dosage of vitamin D is 400 to 600 IU daily.

Vitamin B helps reduce levels of homocysteine, an amino acid linked to cognitive impairment associated with AD. Three B vitamins, folate (natural sources)/folic acid (supplements), B6, and B12, are essential for cognitive function and to prevent anemia. In an Oxford University study of elders with elevated homocysteine levels and memory problems, supplementation with these three vitamins improved memory and reduced brain atrophy (de Jager et al., 2012; Douaud et al., 2013).

Healthful sources of **folate** include leafy greens, such as broccoli, kale, and spinach. Other sources include beans, peas, citrus fruits, and cantaloupe. The recommended dietary allowance (RDA) for folic acid in adults is 400 µg per day, or the equivalent of a bowl of fortified breakfast cereal or a large leafy green salad topped with beans, asparagus, avocadoes, and sliced oranges and sprinkled with peanuts.

Vitamin B6 is found in green vegetables and beans, whole grains, bananas, nuts, and sweet potatoes. The RDA for adults up to 50 years of age is 1.3 mg per day. For adults older than 50, the RDA is 1.5 mg for women and 1.7 mg for men. A half-cup of brown rice meets the recommended amount (Physician's Committee, 2013). Vitamin B6 can also be found in sunflower seeds, tuna, turkey, chicken, prunes, bananas, and avocados.

Vitamin B12 can be taken in supplement form or consumed from foods, including fortified soymilk and fortified cereals. The average adult needs 2.4 µg per day. Although vitamin B12 can be found in meats and dairy products, absorption from these sources can be limited in the older individual, those with reduced stomach acid, and those taking certain medications (e.g., the diabetes drug metformin and acid blockers). For this reason, it is recommended that B12 supplements be consumed by all individuals older than 50 years. People on plant-based diets or with absorption problems should take vitamin B12 supplements, regardless of age. Vitamin B12 can be found in clams, mackerel, bran, skim milk, swiss cheese, and eggs. Following are the recommended daily amounts for supplements:

- Folic acid: 5 mg
- B6: 25 mg
- B12: 1 mg (some studies say 400 µg)

Iron and Copper

Iron and copper are both necessary for health, but studies have linked excessive iron and copper intake to cognitive problems

(Brewer, 2009; Stankiewicz & Brass, 2009). Most individuals meet the recommended intake of these minerals from everyday foods and do not require supplementation. When choosing a multiple vitamin, it is prudent to favor products that deliver vitamins only. Iron supplements should not be used unless absolutely necessary. The RDA for iron for women older than 50 and for men at any age is 8 mg. For women 19 to 50 years of age, the RDA is 18 mg. The RDA for copper for men and women is 0.9 mg.

Aluminum

If aluminum plays a role in AD, it still remains unclear and controversial. Some researchers have called for caution regarding the intake of aluminum, citing its known neurotoxic potential when taken into the body in more than modest amounts (Kawahara & Kato-Negishi, 2011) and the fact that it has been found in the brains of individuals with AD (Physician's Committee, 2013) Studies in the United Kingdom and France found increased Alzheimer's prevalence in areas where tap water contained higher aluminum concentrations (Rondeau et al., 2009). Some experts argue that there is insufficient evidence to verify that aluminum is a contributor to increased risk of AD. Aluminum can be found in certain brands of baking powder, antacids, certain food products, such as bleached flour and pickles, and antiperspirants.

Antioxidants

Antioxidants, substances that neutralize potentially harmful free radicals (electrically charged molecules of oxygen in the bloodstream that take electrons away from other molecules, causing stress to various tissues), have shown promise at potentially preventing AD and have been the subject of extensive study. Evidence of the benefits of antioxidants has been gained through laboratory research and observation. As mentioned, substances with high antioxidant activity include anthocyanins, beta-carotene, catechins, coenzyme Q10 (CoQ10), flavonoids, lipoic acid (also called alpha lipoic acid), lutein, lycopene, selenium, and vitamins A, C, and E. Fish oils and other substances also have antioxidant properties.

Studies investigating lipoic acid and fish oil to slow the progression of AD have shown promise. Lipoic acid is unique as an antioxidant because it functions in water as well as fat, unlike the more common antioxidants vitamins C and vitamin E, and it appears to be able to recycle antioxidants such as vitamin C and glutathione after they have been used up. Glutathione is an important antioxidant that helps the body eliminate potentially harmful substances. Lipoic acid increases the formation of glutathione. The recommended dose of lipoic acid is one 50- to 300-mg oral capsule once or twice daily. Lipoic acid can be found in red meat, spinach, broccoli, potatoes, yams, carrots, beets, and yeast. Lipoic acid supplements can cause some side effects, including potentially lowering blood glucose levels, upset stomach, numbness or tingly feelings, dizziness, tiredness, headache, muscle cramps, and, mild skin rash.

Anthocyanins are the pigments in brightly colored berries. They can be found in plums, cherries, cranberries, blueberries, bananas, red cabbage, grapes, pomegranate, and kidney and black beans. Anthocyanins give cherries their bright red color and possess anti-inflammatory properties that could work like pain medications such as rofecoxib (Vioxx) and celecoxib (Celebrex) but without the nasty side effects. Cherries do not irritate the stomach the way manufactured drugs do, and they contain compounds that keep platelets in the blood from clumping together.

Quercetin, another antioxidant and flavonoid, is found in abundance in the skins of apples. It has been found to protect the brain from damage associated with AD and other neurodegenerative disorders. Some studies have suggested that eating apples may also help reduce the risk of cancer. Alternative foods for the brain, including capers, a common ingredient in Mediterranean cuisine, lovage, red onion, and berries such as cherries, raspberries, and cranberries, contain quercetin in lower amounts.

The following includes information about a variety of other substances with antioxidant properties. Information on these herbs and nutrients was taken from several sources, including "Common dietary supplements for cognitive health" in Aging Health (Gestuvo & Hung, 2012) and a web page on dietary supplements by NCCAM-NIH (2013).

Fish Oil. The benefit of fish oil seems to come from the omega-3 fatty acids that it contains. The body does not produce its own omega-3 fatty acids, nor can the body make them from omega-6 fatty acids, which are common in the Western diet. A lot of research has been done on EPA and DHA (docosahexaenoic acid), two types of omega-3 acids that are often included in fish oil supplements. DHA is found in the meat of cold-water fish, including mackerel, herring, tuna, halibut, salmon, cod liver, whale blubber, and seal blubber. Fish oil has been shown to improve brain functioning, including in individuals with AD, and lower triglyceride levels, which is important because dyslipidemia is another risk factor for AD.

Information on the recommended dose varies; some sources recommend a minimum of 500 mg (0.5 g) of EPA with DHA a day for healthy people and 1000 mg (1 g) a day for those with known heart disease. Others recommend 5 g of fish oil containing 169 to 563 mg of EPA and 72 to 312 mg of DHA. DHA should not be used in amounts greater than 3 g per day. The best fish oil supplements contain 280 mg of DHA and 120 mg of EPA per capsule.

Whereas omega-3s are generally safe for most adults at low to moderate doses, they do have some side effects and pose some safety concerns. Certain fish oil supplements may contain high levels of mercury, pesticides, or PCBs. However, most supplements do not appear to contain these substances. Fish oils containing DHA can thin the blood and increase the risk for bleeding and bruising and cause minor gastrointestinal problems, including nausea, diarrhea, heartburn, indigestion, intestinal gas, and abdominal bloating. Fish oils containing DHA can cause a prolonged fishy taste, belching, nosebleeds, and loose stools. Taking them with meals can often decrease these side effects. If fish oil supplements are taken in high doses, they can interact with certain medications, including blood thinners and drugs used for high blood pressure.

Asian Ginseng. Asian ginseng is an herb with potential effects on insulin resistance, cancer, and AD. It is regarded as an adaptogen, a substance that strengthens and normalizes body functions, helping the body deal with various forms of stress. Ginseng may shorten the time it takes to bounce back from illness or surgery, especially for older individuals. Although Asian ginseng has been widely studied, research results do not conclusively support the health claims associated with use of the herb. The recommended dose is 1000 mg a day or less.

Short-term use of ginseng at recommended doses appears to be safe for most people; however, some sources suggest that prolonged use might cause side effects. Common side effects include headaches, sleep problems, and gastrointestinal problems. Other potential side effects include breast tenderness, menstrual irregularities, and high blood pressure. Asian ginseng may lower levels of blood sugar. Diabetics should use extra caution with this herb, especially if they are using medicines to lower blood sugar or are taking other herbs.

Cat's Claw. Cat's claw is a vine herb native to South America. Its bark and root are used to make teas and powdered supplements. No conclusive studies have proven whether cat's claw can prevent or slow AD, but there are indications that it may help. The exact mechanism is not understood, but the National Institute on Aging funded a study that looked at how cat's claw may affect the brain. Findings may point to new avenues for research in AD treatment. The recommended dose is 60 to 100 mg daily.

Few side effects have been reported for cat's claw when it is taken at recommended dosages. Though rare, side effects may include headaches, dizziness, and vomiting. Women who are pregnant or trying to become pregnant should avoid using cat's claw because it has been used to prevent and abort pregnancy. Cat's claw may stimulate the immune system, but it is unclear whether the herb is safe for people with immune disorders. It may interfere with controlling blood pressure during or after surgery.

Grape Seed Extract. The National Center for Complementary and Alternative Medicine (NCCAM) is studying whether the action of grape seed extract and its components may benefit the heart or help prevent cognitive decline, AD, and other brain disorders. Researchers found that mice treated with grape seed extract had significantly reduced AD-type cognitive deterioration compared with control mice due to the prevention of a molecule, amyloid, forming in the brain, which has been shown to cause AD-type cognitive impairment ("Grape Seed Extract," 2008). More research is underway to investigate whether the same effects can be seen in humans. The recommended dose is 100 to 300 mg per day.

Although grape seed extract is generally well tolerated when taken by mouth and has been used safely for up to 8 weeks in studies, it does have some side effects. These include a dry, itchy scalp; dizziness; headache; high blood pressure; hives; indigestion; and nausea. Interactions between grape seed extract and medicines or other supplements have not been carefully studied.

Coenzyme Q10. Coenzyme Q10, or ubiquinone, is an antioxidant that occurs naturally in the body and is needed for normal cell reactions. Research showed that a synthetic version, called idebenone, did not show effectiveness in preventing or slowing AD. Little is known about what dosage of CoQ10 is considered safe, and there could be harmful effects if too much is taken (NCCAM-NIH, 2013). Dietary supplementation with CoQ10 in mice for one month significantly suppressed brain protein carbonyl levels, which are markers of oxidative damage (Wadsworth et al., 2008). Treatment strategies with antioxidants, including CoQ10, have been proposed for AD because the neurodegenerative process in AD is marked by oxidative damage to the brain. More studies are needed to determine if this sort of treatment is effective in individuals with AD.

The recommended dose of CoQ10 is 50 to 1,200 mg, taken in divided doses by mouth daily. Side effects of CoQ10 are typically mild and brief and generally stop without any treatment needed. Reactions may include nausea, vomiting, stomach upset, heartburn, diarrhea, loss of appetite, skin itching, rash, insomnia, headache, dizziness, itching, irritability, increased light sensitivity of the eyes, fatigue, or flu-like symptoms. This substance also may lower blood sugar levels, blood platelet count, and blood pressure. Organ damage due to lack of oxygen/blood flow during intense exercise has been reported in a study of patients with heart disease, although the specific role of CoQ10 is not clear. Vigorous exercise is often discouraged in people using CoQ10 supplements.

Acetyl-L-carnitine. Acetyl-L-carnitine (ALCAR) is an amino acid (a building block for proteins) that is naturally produced in the body. It helps the body produce energy. It is used for a variety of mental disorders, including AD. ALCAR functions as an antioxidant and promotes the production of glutathione, a free radical scavenger, in cells. ALCAR is a compound acting as an intracellular carrier of acetyl groups across inner mitochondrial membranes and appears to have neuroprotective properties. Recently, it was shown to reduce attention problems in individuals with AD after long-term treatment (Bianchetti et al., 2003). Studies suggest that the vitamin-like nutrient L-carnitine may be able to slow down, or even reverse, brain deterioration. What's more, it may give people the ability to think more clearly and improve memory (Veracity, 2005).

The recommended dose of ALCAR is 500 to 1,500 mg per day. This substance does have some side effects, which may include mild gastrointestinal symptoms, such as nausea, vomiting, and abdominal cramps; headache; and an increase in agitation or restlessness. It should be avoided in individuals with a history of seizure disorder, because it may cause an increase in seizure frequency. Individuals with AD who take ALCAR may exhibit psychiatric disturbances, such as depression and confusion, but it is uncertain whether these effects are due to ALCAR or the disease itself. Some evidence suggests that ALCAR may interfere with thyroid metabolism.

Phosphatidylserine. Phosphatidylserine is a lipid, or fat, that is the primary component of the membranes that surround nerve cells. In AD, nerve cells degenerate for reasons that are not fully understood. Phosphatidylserine may shore up the cell membrane and protect cells from degenerating. The first clinical trials with phosphatidylserine were conducted with a form derived from the brain cells of cows. Some of these trials had promising results. However, most trials were with small samples (Alzheimer's Association, 2014a). Studies ended in the 1990s over concerns about mad cow disease (bovine spongiform encephalopathy), a fatal brain disorder believed to be caused by consuming foods or other products from affected cattle. Phosphatidylserine supplements are now being derived from soy extracts. The FDA has permitted very limited preliminary scientific research using supplements containing very high-quality soy-derived phosphatidylserine, and these studies suggest that this substance may reduce the risk of dementia in older individuals.

The recommended dose of phosphatidylserine is 100 mg three times daily. There is some concern that products made from animal sources could transmit diseases, such as mad cow disease. To date, there are no known cases of humans getting animal diseases from phosphatidylserine supplements, but to be safe, choose supplements that are made from plants. Side effects may include insomnia and stomach upset.

Dehydroepiandrosterone. Dehydroepiandrosterone (DHEA) is a hormone produced normally by the adrenal glands, but the exact function of DHEA in the body is unclear. It is a popular dietary supplement touted as having anti-aging effects. Interest in DHEA supplements was stimulated by findings that levels of the hormone peak between the ages of 20 and 30 and then decrease steadily with age. In addition, some animal studies showed that giving DHEA supplements to older mice improved their memory. However, studies in humans found that DHEA supplements did not improve mental performance or lessen overall severity of AD after six months of treatment (WebMD, 2014). Potential side effects include acne, hair loss, unwanted hair growth, voice deepening, irritability, insomnia, and aggressiveness.

Huperzine A. Huperzine A is a substance purified from a plant called Chinese club moss. Although huperzine A comes from a plant, the product is the result of a lot of laboratory manipulation — it is a highly purified drug. Huperzine A is thought to be beneficial for problems with memory, loss of mental abilities (dementia), and the muscular disorder myasthenia gravis, because it causes an increase in the levels of acetylcholine, which is one of the neurochemicals destroyed too rapidly in individuals with AD.

The recommended dose is 30 to 200 µg of huperzine A twice daily. This substance may lower blood pressure and slow heart rate. Side effects may include nausea, diarrhea, vomiting, sweating, blurred vision, slurred speech, restlessness, loss of appetite, contraction and twitching of muscle fibers, cramping, increased saliva and urine, and inability to control urination.

Vinpocetine. Vinpocetine is a manufactured chemical resembling a substance found in the periwinkle plant *Vinca minor*. It is thought to improve blood flow to the brain and is used for enhancing memory and preventing AD, as well as other conditions that harm learning, memory, and information processing skills as people age. It is not known exactly how vinpocetine works, but it might increase blood flow to the brain and offer some protection for brain cells (neurons) against injury (WebMD, 2014).

The recommended dose is 5 to 10 mg of vinpocetine three times daily. This substance may thin blood and cause more bleeding. It also may cause some side effects, including stomach pain, nausea, sleep disturbances, headache, dizziness, nervousness, and flushing of the face.

One Brain-Healthy Diet: The Mediterranean Diet

Several studies have investigated the association between adherence to the Mediterranean diet and health status and found a significant association between the Mediterranean diet and a reduced risk of major chronic degenerative diseases, including AD (Sofi et al., 2010). Moreover, the Mediterranean diet has been extensively reported to be associated with a favorable health outcome and a better quality of life. A heart-healthy Mediterranean diet is rich in fish, nuts, whole grains, olive oil, and abundant fresh produce. An occasional glass of red wine and square of dark chocolate may also assist in improving the health of the brain.

The Mediterranean diet offers an abundance of food from plant sources, including fruits and vegetables, potatoes, breads and grains, beans, nuts, and seeds. There is an emphasis on a variety of minimally processed and, when possible, seasonally fresh and locally grown foods (which can maximize the health-promoting micronutrient and antioxidant content of these foods). Olive oil is the principal fat, replacing other fats and oils (including butter and margarine). Total fat in the daily diet should range from less than 25% to more than 35% of energy (calories), with saturated fat at no more than 7 to 8% of energy. Other components of this diet include daily consumption of low to moderate amounts of cheese and yogurt (with low-fat and non-fat versions possibly being preferable); twice-a-week consumption of low to moderate amounts of fish and poultry (with fish being favored over poultry); and up to seven eggs per week (including those used in cooking and baking). Fresh fruit should be the typical daily dessert; sweets with a significant amount of sugar (prefer honey) and saturated fat should not be consumed more than a few times a week. Recent research suggests that, if red meat is eaten, it should be limited to a few times a month, at a maximum of 12 to 16 ounces (340–450 g) per month. When the flavor is acceptable, lean versions may be preferable (Greenstein, n.d.).

Moderate consumption of wine, normally drunk with meals, may have some benefits. Quantities should not exceed about one to two glasses per day for men and one glass per day for women. Wine is considered optional and should be avoided when consumption would put the individual or others at risk.

The following reviews the basics of the Mediterranean diet:

1. **Eat lots of vegetables.** From a simple plate of sliced fresh tomatoes drizzled with olive oil and crumbled feta cheese to gorgeous salads, garlicky greens, fragrant soups and stews, healthy pizzas, or oven-roasted medleys, vegetables are vitally important to the fresh tastes and delicious flavors of the Mediterranean diet.

2. **Eat small amounts of lean meats.** If an individual wishes to eat meat, have smaller amounts; e.g., small strips of sirloin in a vegetable sauté, or a dish of pasta garnished with diced prosciutto.

3. **Always eat breakfast.** Start the day with fiber-rich foods, such as fruit and whole grains, which make a person feel full for hours. Layer granola, yogurt, and fruit, or mash half an avocado with a fork and spread it on a slice of whole-grain toast.

4. **Eat seafood twice a week.** Include fish such as tuna, herring, salmon, and sardines, which are rich in omega-3 fatty acids, and shellfish, including mussels, oysters, and clams, which have similar benefits for brain and heart health.

5. **Cook a vegetarian meal one night a week.** Build meals around beans, whole grains, and vegetables, and heighten the flavor with fragrant herbs and spices. Consider increasing to two nights per week as time goes on.

6. **Use good fats.** Include sources of healthy fats in daily meals, especially extra-virgin olive oil, nuts, peanuts, sunflower seeds, olives, and avocados.

7. **Enjoy some dairy products.** Eat Greek or plain yogurt, and try small amounts of a variety of cheeses.

8. **For dessert, eat fresh fruit.** Choose from a wide range of delicious fresh fruits — from fresh figs and oranges

to pomegranates, grapes, and apples. Instead of daily ice cream or cookies, save sweets for a special treat or celebration.

Elements of a Heart-Healthy Diet

Eating a low-cholesterol, low-sodium diet will improve heart functioning, reduce arteriosclerotic cardiovascular disease, and improve the brain health while lowering the risk for AD. Although you might know that eating certain foods can increase your heart disease risk, it's often tough to change your eating habits. Whether an individual has experienced years of unhealthy eating or simply wants to fine-tune his or her diet, the following eight heart-healthy diet tips can help. The following list and tables were taken from Mayo Clinic, "Heart-Healthy Diet: 8 Steps to Prevent Heart Disease" (2012a).

1. **Control portion size.** The amount a person eats is just as important as what type of food is eaten. Overloading the plate, taking seconds, and eating until full or even stuffed can lead to eating more calories, fat, and cholesterol than a person should. Portions served in restaurants are often more than needed. Keep track of the number of servings eaten and use proper serving sizes to help control intake. Eating more low-calorie, nutrient-rich foods, such as fruits and vegetables, and less of high-calorie, high-sodium foods, such as refined, processed, or fast foods, can improve one's diet and be beneficial for the heart as well as weight. A serving size is a specific amount of food, defined by common measurements such as cups, ounces, or pieces. For example, one serving of pasta is a half cup, or about the size of a hockey puck. A serving of meat, fish, or chicken is 2 to 3 ounces, or about the size and thickness of a deck of cards.

2. **Eat more vegetables and fruits.** Vegetables and fruits are excellent sources of vitamins and minerals. They can be low in calories and rich in dietary fiber and contain substances that may help prevent cardiovascular disease.

107

Eating more fruits and vegetables may help a person eat less high-fat foods, such as meat, cheese, and snack foods. Featuring vegetables and fruits in an individual's diet can be easy. Keep vegetables washed, cut, and in the refrigerator for quick snacks. Keep fruit in a bowl in the kitchen so it is easier to eat than non-nutritious snacks. Choose recipes that have vegetables or fruits as the main ingredient, such as a vegetable stir-fry or salads containing fresh fruit.

3. **Select whole grains.** Whole grains are good sources of fiber and other nutrients that help regulate blood pressure

Fruits and Vegetables to Choose
• Fresh or frozen vegetables and fruits
• Low-sodium canned vegetables
• Canned fruit packed in juice or water
Fruits and Vegetables to Limit or Avoid
• Coconut
• Vegetables with creamy sauces or gravy
• Fried or breaded vegetables
• Canned fruit packed in heavy syrup
• Frozen fruit with sugar added

and heart health. Increase the amount of whole grains in a heart-healthy diet by making simple substitutions for refined grain products or try a new whole grain, such as whole-grain couscous, quinoa, or barley. Another good additive to the diet is ground flaxseed. Flaxseeds are small brown seeds that are high in fiber and omega-3 fatty acids, which can lower blood cholesterol. A person can grind the seeds in a coffee grinder or food processor and stir a teaspoon of them into yogurt, applesauce, or hot cereal.

4. **Limit unhealthy fats and cholesterol.** Limit saturated and trans fats — an important step to reduce blood

cholesterol and lower the risk of coronary artery disease, as well as AD. A high blood cholesterol level can lead to the buildup of plaques in the arteries, also known as atherosclerosis, which can increase a person's risk of heart attack and stroke. The American Heart Association offers these guidelines for how much fat and cholesterol to include in a heart-healthy diet:

The best way to reduce saturated and trans fats in a diet is to limit the amount of solid fats (e.g., butter, margarine

Type of Fat	Recommendation
Saturated fat	Less than 7% of total daily calories, or less than 14 g of saturated fat if following a 2,000-calorie-a-day diet
Trans fat	Less than 1% of total daily calories, or less than 2 g of trans fat if following a 2,000-calorie-a-day diet
Cholesterol	Less than 300 mg a day for healthy adults; less than 200 mg a day for adults with high levels of LDL ("bad") cholesterol or those who are taking cholesterol-lowering medication

and shortening), which are often added to food when cooking and serving. It can also help to trim fat off meat or choose lean meats, with less than 10% fat. Use low-fat substitutions when possible. For example, top a baked potato with salsa or low-fat yogurt rather than butter, or use low-sugar fruit spread on toast instead of margarine.

Check the food labels of some cookies, crackers, and chips — many of these snacks, even those labeled "reduced fat," may be made with oils containing trans fats. One clue that a food has some trans fat in it is the phrase "partially hydrogenated" in the ingredient list. When using fats, choose monounsaturated fats, such as olive or canola oil. Polyunsaturated fats, found in nuts and seeds, also are good choices for a heart-healthy diet. When used in place of saturated fats, monounsaturated and polyunsaturated fats may help lower total blood cholesterol. However, moderation is essential: Remember that all types of fat are high in calories.

5. **Choose low-fat protein sources.** Lean meat, poultry, and fish; low-fat dairy products; and egg whites or egg

Fats to Choose
• Olive oil
• Canola oil
• Margarine that is free of trans fats
• Cholesterol-lowering margarines, such as Benecol, Promise Activ, or Smart Balance

Fats to Limit or Avoid
• Butter
• Lard
• Bacon fat
• Gravy
• Cream sauce
• Nondairy creamers
• Hydrogenated margarine and shortening
• Cocoa butter, found in chocolate
• Coconut, palm, cottonseed, and palm-kernel oils

substitutes are some of the best sources of protein. Care should be taken to choose lower-fat options, such as skim milk rather than whole milk, and skinless chicken breasts rather than fried chicken patties. Fish is another good alternative to high-fat meats, and certain types of fish are rich in omega-3 fatty acids, which can lower blood fats called triglycerides. Cold-water fish, such as salmon, mackerel, and herring, have the highest amounts of omega-3 fatty acids. Other sources are flaxseed, walnuts, soybeans, and canola oil. Legumes (beans, peas, and lentils) also are good sources of protein and contain less fat and no cholesterol, making them good substitutes for meat. Substituting plant protein for animal protein (for example, a soy or bean burger for a hamburger) will reduce fat and cholesterol intake.

Proteins to Choose
• Low-fat dairy products, such as skim or low-fat (1%) milk, yogurt, and cheese
• Egg whites or egg substitutes
• Fish, especially fatty, cold-water fish, such as salmon
• Skinless poultry
• Legumes
• Soybeans and soy products; e.g., soy burgers and tofu
• Lean ground meats

Proteins to Limit or Avoid
• Full-fat milk and other dairy products
• Organ meats, such as liver
• Egg yolks
• Fatty and marbled meats
• Spareribs
• Cold cuts
• Hot dogs and sausages
• Bacon
• Fried or breaded meats

6. Reduce sodium. Eating a lot of sodium can contribute to high blood pressure, a risk factor for cardiovascular disease. Reducing sodium is an important part of a heart-healthy diet. The Department of Agriculture recommends the following:

- Healthy adults have no more than 2,300 mg of sodium a day (about a teaspoon)
- Older individuals (51 years and older), African Americans, and people with high blood pressure, diabetes, or chronic kidney disease have no more than 1,500 mg of sodium a day

Although reducing the amount of salt added to food at the table or while cooking is a good first step, much of the sodium eaten comes from canned or processed foods, such as soups and frozen dinners. Eating fresh foods and making soups and stews from scratch can reduce the amount of sodium in the diet. If the convenience of canned soups and prepared meals is preferred, look for food choices with reduced sodium. Be wary of foods that claim to be lower in sodium because they are seasoned with sea salt instead of regular table salt: Sea salt has the same nutritional value as regular salt. Another way to reduce salt is to choose condiments carefully: Many are available in reduced-sodium versions, and salt substitutes can add flavor to food with less sodium.

Low-Salt Items to Choose
• Herbs and spices
• Salt substitutes
• Reduced-salt canned soups or prepared meals
• Reduced-salt versions of condiments, such as reduced-salt soy sauce and reduced-salt ketchup

High-Salt Items to Avoid
• Table salt
• Canned soups and prepared foods, such as frozen dinners
• Tomato juice
• Soy sauce

7. **Plan ahead: Create daily menus.** Plan meals and know what foods to choose for a heart-healthy diet and which ones to limit. Create daily menus using the six strategies previously discussed. When selecting foods for a meal or a snack, emphasize vegetables, fruits, and whole grains. Choose lean protein sources and limit high-fat and salty foods. Watch portion sizes, and add variety to the menu.

8. **Allow an occasional treat.** Allow an indulgence every now and then. A candy bar or handful of potato chips won't derail the heart-healthy diet if most of the time a person follows a healthy diet.

Seven Foods for Preventing Alzheimer's Disease

The following foods may help prevent AD (Breslau, n.d.).

1. **Walnuts (as well as almonds, pecans, hazelnuts).** Walnuts might be small in size, but they pack a big nutritional punch. They are high in omega-3 fatty acids, the good kind of fat the brain needs. They also contain vitamin E and flavonoids, which can help protect the brain.

2. Salmon (as well as mackerel, sardines, other fatty fish). As mentioned earlier in this book, fatty fish like salmon is also high in omega-3s and can lower blood levels of beta-amyloid, a protein thought to play a role in increasing risks for developing AD. Eating 8 ounces of fish per week is recommended — fresh fish is best, but taking a fish oil supplement may be equivalent in offering prevention from AD.

3. Berries. Berries contain polyphenols, a type of antioxidant that helps stop inflammation and allows brain cells to work better. A study found that berries can reverse slow-downs in the brain's ability to process information. A cup of strawberries, blueberries, or cranberries a day helps decrease an individual's risks for developing AD.

4. Spinach (as well as kale, other leafy greens). Green leafy vegetables are full of antioxidants and fiber and should be a diet staple. In a national study, women in their 60s who ate more green leafy vegetables did better over time than their non–greens-eating counterparts on memory, verbal, and other tests. What's more, new studies show that high levels of vitamin C, which is found in spinach, may help with dementia prevention.

5. Turmeric. Several studies have shown that turmeric, the spice used in curries, and its main active component, curcumin, can help prevent Alzheimer's. One UCLA study found that vitamin D3, taken with curcumin, may help the immune system get rid of the amino acids that form the plaque in the brain associated with the development of AD.

6. Coffee. Some studies indicate that people older than 65 who drank three cups of coffee a day (i.e., had higher blood levels of caffeine) developed AD two to four years later than their counterparts with lower caffeine levels, and that caffeine had a positive impact even in older adults who were already showing early signs of Alzheimer's.

7. **Chocolate.** Compelling research already shows that dark chocolate, which contains flavonoids, can help combat heart disease, but flavonoids also help slow down the effects of dementia. In an Italian study, older adults who had mild symptoms of dementia drank cocoa with high, medium, and low amounts of flavonoids. Those who consumed high amounts outperformed those who consumed low doses on cognitive tests. A healthy choice is dark chocolate that has a 70% or higher cocoa content.

Lifestyle Strategies

There are other factors aside from diet that must be followed to provide the best strategy for preventing AD:

- Not smoking (or stopping smoking)
- Being physically and mentally active
- Obtaining quality sleep
- Stress management
- Properly treating or preventing chronic diseases and conditions, such as hypertension, high blood cholesterol, diabetes, obesity, and depression

Physical Activity

Studies show that a person who is physically active is less likely to experience a decline in his or her mental function and less likely to develop AD. Exercising several times a week for 30 to 60 minutes may:

- Keep thinking, reasoning, and learning skills sharp in healthy individuals
- Improve memory, reasoning, judgment, and thinking skills (cognitive function) for individuals with mild AD or MCI
- Delay the start of AD for those at risk of developing the disease or slow the progression of the disease

Physical activity seems to have positive impacts on the brain aside from just keeping a person's blood flowing. It also increases chemicals that protect the brain and tend to counter some of the natural reduction in brain connections that occurs with aging (Mayo Clinic, 2014a). Endurance exercises increase the effect of a regulatory metabolic compound, peroxisome proliferator-activated receptor-gamma coactivator 1 alpha, in the muscles of mice, which boosts production of the FNDC5 gene. This has a knock-on effect of switching on genes that increase the expression of a brain-protective protein, brain-derived neurotrophic factor, in the hippocampus, a part of the brain involved in learning and memory (Paddock, 2013). Performing exercise routinely on a daily basis for an average of 30 to 50 minutes is recommended — the more, the better. At a minimum, one should exercise three to five days a week for at least 30 consecutive minutes. Walking, running, cycling, swimming, dancing, or any activity that keeps a person in continuous motion and increases the heart rate is beneficial, as long as the individual can physically tolerate the exercise regimen.

Brain Exercise

Exercise the brain daily: Keep the brain active by learning something new. The more diverse the learning activities, the better for brain health and preventing AD. Here are some suggestions. Brain games are described in more detail in the following sections.

- Stay curious and involved — commit to lifelong learning
- Read, write, and work crosswords or other puzzles
- Attend lectures and plays
- Enroll in courses at the local adult education center, community college, or other community resource
- Enroll in dance classes: Learn different dances (to challenge the brain as well as the body and assist in improving balance and gait)

- Play games
  - » Sudoku
  - » Crossword puzzles
  - » Word find games

- Garden

- Try memory exercises
  - » Memorize the state capitols or poems
  - » Play games such as the picnic memory game
  - » Neighborhood watch: Learn the cars that live in the neighborhood and watch for different cars; write down the model of the car, the color, and the tag/ license plate

Exercising the brain may help prevent AD or slow down its progress, and one way to do this is by playing certain types of games. The following are suggested brain games — the more novel, the better. Learn information in ways that are different from the usual; for example, if your interests are in nursing, learn something mechanical. The following list was adapted from "Brain Games for Alzheimer's" (Mayne, 2013).

- **Crossword Puzzles.** Crossword puzzles are intellectually stimulating and require several mental activities, including word skills, geometrical skills, and logic. Consider increasing the complexity of the crossword puzzles after easier ones are mastered. They are easy to find and inexpensive.

- **Word Find Games.** Word find, or word search, games that involve hunting, comparing, spelling, and logic can be mentally stimulating. These games can be found in magazines and newspapers, and there are entire books devoted to word find games. Also consider 3D games, in which the individual must see patterns within patterns.

- **Scrabble and Other Word Games.** Scrabble requires various forms of processing letters, creating words, and generally thinking, which exercises the brain. In addition to the logic of space and placement, spelling, and rational thinking, Scrabble also provides opportunities for socializing. Being a part of a group that plays Scrabble routinely may help alleviate loneliness and depression. A daily game of Scrabble will also help keep the aging mind sharp and give the person something to look forward to every day.

- **Trivia Games.** Trivia games like Trivial Pursuit, Jeopardy, and Family Feud may help stimulate brain function. Some of these games are geared toward familiar information for the generation of adults playing the game; i.e., providing questions and answers from the person's younger days. Trivia games can be played with groups of friends or online.

- **Other Games to Stimulate and Exercise the Brain.** Many games stimulate the brain and keep it active, including strategy games, such as Sudoku, checkers, and chess. Card games can provide a combination of logic, planning, and social skills. Even solitaire may help keep a person's mind focused and sharp. Video and computer games can also be stimulating brain activities to help prevent AD.

Staying Socially Active

Research has shown that leisure activities that combine physical, mental, and social activity are the most likely to prevent dementia. In a study of 800 men and women 75 years and older, those who were more physically active, more mentally active, or more socially engaged had a lower risk of developing dementia than their peers who were more isolated, and those who combined these activities did even better (Alzheimer's Association, 2014g). Other research found that sports, cultural activities, emotional support, and close personal relationships together appear to have a protective effect against dementia. Stay socially engaged in activities that stimulate the mind and body through activities such as the following:

- Stay active in the workplace

- Volunteer in community groups and causes
- Join social clubs, square dancing groups, or other socially active groups
- Travel

Sleep

Whiteman (2013) reported on research on sleep and AD done at the Johns Hopkins Bloomberg School of Health. Previous research had linked disturbed sleep to cognitive impairment in older individuals, with individuals with AD having been shown to spend more time awake and have higher levels of fragmented sleep, compared with those who do not have the disorder. Sleep patterns had previously been linked to beta-amyloid plaques, and changes in beta-amyloid levels may be regulated by sleep-wake patterns. The researchers used brain imaging to study sleep duration in people with no dementia and found that a shorter overall night's sleep duration and poor sleep quality were linked to increased beta-amyloid build-up, which is one of the key features of AD. Research into beta-amyloid deposition in the brain has suggested quality sleep "detoxes" the brain by flushing out the waste products of neural activity. Researchers further have determined that late-life sleep disturbance can be treated, and interventions to improve sleep or maintain healthy sleep among older adults may help prevent or slow AD to the extent that poor sleep promotes AD onset and progression. Causes of interrupted sleep may include:

- Snoring or obstructive sleep apnea
- Insomnia (trouble getting to sleep, staying asleep, or waking up early)
- Nocturia (getting up several times a night to urinate)
- Restless leg syndrome
- Cognitive impairments, which cause vivid dreams, nightmares, or "sundowning" (increased confusion and agitation, often at night, in an individual who has dementia)

Some people begin taking a sleep aid to assist in obtaining adequate sleep. However, sleep agents should be used with caution, because they may cause an older person to fall or be more confused. Some sleep agents disrupt a person's REM sleep so that he or she does not dream. The REM sleep (dream sleep) is very important, because this is the restorative sleep that helps detoxify the brain.

CHAPTER 7

SLOWING ALZHEIMER'S DISEASE

ALZHEIMER'S DISEASE IS A PROGRESSIVE DISORDER, BUT INDIVIDUALS MAY BE ABLE TO SLOW THE PROGRESSION THROUGH VARIOUS TECHNIQUES. THIS CHAPTER PRESENTS STRATEGIES TO HELP SLOW THE COGNITIVE DECLINE AND DIMINISH OR PREVENT BEHAVIORAL ISSUES.

Although there is no cure for AD, the mainstay of therapy is aimed at temporarily slowing the progression of the disease, slowing the symptoms, and improving independence as well as quality of life for those with the disease and their caregivers. There are certain medications and lifestyle changes that can assist in slowing the progression of the disease. This chapter begins with a discussion of medications currently used to treat and slow the progression of the disease. However, medications are not the only treatments that have been shown to slow AD progression. Other strategies include mental stimulation, developing a routine and establishing a sense of familiarity, and dietary supplements of vitamins and herbs. Some of the treatments discussed in this chapter are the same as or similar to those discussed earlier in this book for preventing and treating AD and other forms of dementia.

Medications

Treatment for AD consists of slowing the progression of the disease, improving quality of life, and managing the problems caused by AD. There are several different types of medications used to treat the associated memory loss, behavior changes, sleep problems, and the other symptoms of AD. A word of caution is that all medications used in the management of dementia, including AD, can have side effects, which can be even more pronounced in frail elders. These drugs are discussed below and in **Table 7-1**, with recommended dosages for older adults, as well as their side effects.

Cholinesterase Inhibitors and N-Methyl-D-Aspartate

As noted earlier in this book, there are two classes of drugs approved by the FDA for treating AD: cholinesterase inhibitors and NMDA. In the brains of individuals with AD, acetylcholine is destroyed too rapidly, making it difficult for the signals to be transmitted along the neural pathway. Cholinesterase inhibitors are used to slow the destruction (and thus the progression) of AD and to help improve cognitive symptoms. These medications work by preventing the breakdown of a chemical messenger in the brain called acetylcholine, which is important for learning, memory, and attention. There are three cholinesterase inhibitors approved for the treatment of AD: donepezil (Aricept), which is indicated and approved to treat the mild, moderate, and severe stages of Alzheimer's, and rivastigmine (Exelon) and galantamine (Razadyne), which are indicated and approved to treat the mild to moderate stages of AD. Rivastigmine is also approved to treat Parkinson's disease dementia. Side effects associated with the use of the cholinesterase inhibitors include nausea, vomiting, diarrhea, weight loss, and dizziness.

The second class of drugs approved by the FDA to treat Alzheimer's disease is NMDA. There is only one medication in this class: memantine (Namenda), which works by regulating the amount of another chemical messenger in the brain called glutamate. Glutamate is made in excess in the moderate and late stages of AD, which causes interference with information retrieval and memory, as well as behavioral problems. Memantine is indicated and approved by the FDA for treating the moderate to severe stages of AD and works by binding with the excessive glutamate. Side effects can include dizziness, confusion, headache, constipation, nausea, and agitation. Because memantine and cholinesterase inhibitors work on different chemicals in the brain, they are often used in combination.

Other Medications

As previously discussed, there are other medications commonly used in caring for individuals with AD to help manage the behavioral and psychiatric symptoms, including hallucinations, agitation, and sleep problems. However, none of these medications are indicated or approved by the FDA to treat dementia, including AD. Nonetheless, these medications are commonly used and can be found in current literature discussing treatment of behavioral problems exhibited by individuals with dementia. The three main classes of medications include antidepressants, which treat depression, anxiolytics, which treat anxiety and restlessness, and antipsychotics, which treat hallucinations, delusions, agitation, and aggression.

Antidepressants. Depression is common in individuals with AD and other types of dementia. Often, antidepressant medications are used to treat this problem. The class of drugs most commonly prescribed in the elderly population is SSRI antidepressants because of their therapeutic efficacy and favorable side-effect profile (Salzman, Schneider, & Alexopoulos, 2000). They are highly selective in treating depression symptoms, are well known for their benign interaction, and are equally effective to and far safer than treatment with antipsychotic medications (Rosack, 2002): Antidepressants have been shown to be just as effective as an antipsychotic for calming agitation and treating psychotic symptoms in older individuals with dementia (Chow, Pollock, & Milgram, 2007). There are other classes of antidepressant medications, but the SSRIs are the class of choice in the geriatric population.

Anxiolytics. Anxiety is another common problem in individuals with dementia. Anxiolytics are a class of anti-anxiety medications used to treat this problem in those with dementia. They work by calming and relaxing a person and may be prescribed in conjunction with other medications to relieve anxiety symptoms or slow the progression of dementia (Masterman, 2003; eHow, 2010). Anxiolytics are good agents to use when a confused individual is unable to be consoled, redirected, or calmed and there is a potential for injury to self or others. They can produce side effects such as sleepiness, fainting, dizziness, blurred vision, confusion, and potential falls due to their effects on balance. There are risks for use of this class if prescribed in high doses, and there are potential interactions with alcohol or other drugs, including depression of brain functioning, can cause slowed respirations and potentially cause a person to stop breathing. Anxiolytics should be used cautiously but may be necessary when an individual is unable to function and has a poor quality of life due to anxiety, paranoia, or extreme delusions.

Antipsychotics. Antipsychotics are not indicated for the treatment of AD, but they are commonly used in individuals with dementia to treat hallucinations, delusions, or extreme "sundowning" behaviors. Antipsychotic medications may decrease the psychosis or agitated behaviors associated with dementia by calming the racing thoughts, paranoia, and agitation, allowing the person to interact with others, follow a routine, and be as independent as possible. This class of medications must not be used as a chemical restraint — using a medication to quiet and sedate an unruly person. Antipsychotic medications may be used to enhance quality of life for an individual who exhibits distressing and agitated behaviors that endanger him or her and/or others.

The benefits for using this type of medication must be weighed against the associated risks. It is important to note that medical problems may occur in older individuals who take antipsychotics, which may include an increased risk of strokes and death in individuals suffering from dementia, worsening of diabetes, worsening of cholesterol problems, and increased risk for falls. Antipsychotics currently have a "black box" warning issued by the FDA regarding their use in older people with dementia because of the increased risk of death. There is a push to decrease or stop the use of antipsychotic medications in elders because of these associated adverse effects. Antipsychotic medications can also cause dystonia: abnormal, repetitious, involuntary movements, such as constant tongue protrusion, constant chewing, rocking motions, and pill rolling. If an individual develops dystonic movements, all medications use must be re-evaluated to determine if continued use is in the person's best interest. Appropriate laboratory monitoring is required with the use of all of the antipsychotic medications and should include tests to monitor liver and kidney functioning, tests of glucose and hemoglobin A1c to monitor status of diabetes, and cholesterol panels at least every 6 months.

Other Medications. Additional medications can be used in the management of the symptoms of AD and other dementias. Anticonvulsants have been used to manage behavioral problems in individuals with dementia. The most commonly used drug in this class is valproic acid (Depakote), which has been used to treat epilepsy, bipolar disorder, and migraine headaches. Psychiatrists observed that valproic acid had certain side effects, including calming of anxious behaviors. It began to be used for these effects on mood and behavior in individuals with behavioral problems.

As described in Chapter 3, valproic acid dampens the speed and frequency with which neurons fire. In addition to assisting in managing anxiety, agitation, and psychotic behaviors in individuals with dementia, scientists also think that valproic acid may inhibit the development of the plaques and tangles in the brains of people with AD (Peterson, 2004). This medication should be used cautiously because it has the potential to cause sedation, falls, and orthostatic hypotension. There is a "black box" warning for liver damage, and people taking this medication must undergo routine monitoring of liver function and drug levels to monitor for and prevent toxicity. Be aware that, for dementia, the level of valproic acid in an individual's blood does not need to be in the therapeutic range, since it is not being used to treat seizures.

Table 7-1. Medications Used to Treat Alzheimer's Disease

Medication Class	Medication and Suggested Dosing in Elders	Potential Side Effects
Cholinesterase inhibitors*	Donepezil (Aricept) • 5 mg daily for 30 days, then 10 mg daily • If higher dose needed: 23 mg daily after the individual has been on 10 mg daily for minimum of 3 months Rivastigmine (Exelon) • Start at 1.5 mg bid for 2 weeks, then 3 mg bid for 2 weeks, then 4.5 mg bid, then 6 mg bid (max. dose, 12 mg/day) • Patch is available: 4.6 mg/24 hours; change once a day, then 9.5 mg/24 hours • If a higher dose is needed: 13.3 mg/24 hours patch daily after the person has been on 9.5 mg/24 hours for minimum of 3 months Galantamine (Razadyne) • 4 mg bid, increase every 4 weeks until reaching 12 mg bid	Most common problems are loss of appetite, nausea, vomiting, abdominal pain, and diarrhea
N-methyl-D-aspartate receptor antagonists†	Memantine (Namenda) • Titration: Start at 5 mg daily for 7 days, then 5 mg bid for 7 days, then 5 mg in morning, 10 mg in evening for 7 days, then 10 mg bid	Sedation, constipation, dizziness, headache, and pain
Antidepressants: SSRIs	Bupropion (Wellbutrin) • 75–100 mg qd or bid Duloxetine (Cymbalta) • 20–60 mg qd Escitalopram (Lexapro) • 5–20 mg qd Fluoxetine (Prozac) • 10–20 mg qd	Weight gain, dizziness, somnolence, insomnia, decreased libido, tremors, akathesia, tremors, nervousness, sweating, and various GI and sexual disturbances

Antidepressants: SSRIs (continued)	Paroxetine (Paxil)
	  • 10–40 mg qd
	Paroxetine CR (Paxil CR)
	  • 12.5–37.5 mg qd
	Sertraline (Zoloft)
	  • 25–50 mg qd
	Venlafaxine XR (Effexor XR)
	  • 37.5–150.0 mg qd
		Sedation, falls, orthostatic hypotension, and increased confusion

Anxiolytics‡	Alprazolam (Xanax)
	  • 0.25–0.5 mg every 6–8 hours as needed
	Clonazepam (Klonipin)
	  • 0.125–2.0 mg every 12 hours as needed
	  • Has a long half-life
	Clorazepapte (Tranxene)
	  • 75–15.0 mg every 8 hours as needed
	Lorazepam (Ativan)
	  • 0.5–2 mg every 6–8 hours as needed
	  • Has the shortest half-life and is the drug of choice in elders with dementia if an anxiolytic is necessary	

*Indicated by the FDA for treatment of early, middle, and late stages of AD.
†Indicated by the FDA for treatment of middle and late stages of AD.
‡Indicated by the FDA for treatment of anxiety symptoms; not recommended for routine use.
bid = twice a day, qd = once a day

Antioxidants and Herbal Supplements

Antioxidants and herbal supplements may help prevent or slow the progression of AD. A lengthy discussion of antioxidants and herbal supplements is presented in Chapter 6. Below is a short list of some substances that may help slow the course of AD:

- Huperzine A to slow memory loss. An active ingredient in the Chinese herb club moss, huperzine A is purported to block the breakdown of acetylcholine, the neurotransmitter important for memory (Phillips, 2007). Recommended dosage is 30 mcg twice a day.

- Phosphatidylserine to boost mental capacity. This substance helps regenerate the outside layer of neurons, reversing the chronological age of these cells by as much as 12 years, and improves mental capacity in people with AD. The recommended dose is 300 mg per day divided into three doses taken with meals (Phillips, 2007).

- Vitamin B to prevent memory loss: Large daily doses of B vitamins may protect vulnerable populations from the brain shrinkage and memory loss associated with AD. Normally, the brain shrinks as people age (about 0.5% per year). In individuals with MCI, this shrinkage takes place twice as fast as usual, and in people with AD, shrinkage happens four times as fast as usual. High daily dose of three B vitamins: folic acid (0.8 mg), vitamin B6 (20 mg), and vitamin B12 (0.5 mg), over the course of two years was found to halt that memory loss (Gutierrez, 2013).

- Vitamin E to regenerate brain cells. Vitamin E helps shield neurons from free radicals, which are the unstable molecules that can damage brain cells. It can also help regenerate the neurons where neurotransmitters, chemicals that relay the messages from one neuron to another, enter. Individuals with AD should take 2000 IU a day of the d-alpha-tocopherol form of the nutrient, which is the most effective (Phillips, 2007).

Mental Stimulation

A growing body of research indicates that stimulating the brain has the power to slow the progression of AD, particularly in the early stages. One study found that healthy elderly adults who were mentally active were 2.6 times less likely to develop dementia that those who were not (Bennett et al., 2012). A person in the early stages of AD should be encouraged to participate in activities that engage the mind that he or she finds pleasurable, such as reading, writing, playing the piano, working crosswords or puzzle books, playing games like chess, or learning a language (Scott, n.d.).

Local senior centers and adult day care programs may offer stimulating activities, including group reminiscent therapy, storytelling, music, art, and games. Some research suggests that activities are especially protective when they involve socializing with other people. Healthy people who interact with others tend to have fewer memory problems than those who are more reclusive. If assistance with household duties is needed or a caregiver stays with an individual who has early-stage AD, avoid relieving the person of all customary chores and responsibilities. Participating in daily chores can be a form of mental workout and increase the person's independence, which in turn prevents or improves depression and anxiety (Scott, n.d.).

It is important that an individual with AD engages in pleasurable activities and avoids those that may cause stress. For example, if he or she finds using a computer frustrating because of existing cognitive declines, it may be more beneficial to encourage the person to perform mental activities that are more familiar. Also, avoid formal mental "exercises" or memory drills, which may cause more stress, thus worsening the symptoms of AD (Scott, n.d.).

Whereas social activity can be beneficial in providing mental stimulation, overstimulation through too much social activity can be stressful. Outings are best when they are low key, such as small dinners as opposed to loud parties. Limit time out to no more than 2 hours at a time so as not to tire the person.

Helping a person with AD to continue engaging in some of his or her usual tasks, such as housework and bill paying, can provide mental stimulation and help maintain independence for as long as possible. This has the added benefits of reducing stress and slowing further decline. Simplifying the living environment and providing the tools to boost the person's existing memory will help make this possible. Consider minimizing or streamlining tasks that may be more difficult due to a person's declining mental and physical state. For example, arrange for electronic bill paying, hire a lawn service, or enlist a neighbor or church member to handle laundry. Help the person with AD keep his or her home free of piled-up newspapers, old mail, and other clutter. Look into electronic reminder systems, note-keeping systems, or commercially available tools that can help to prop up a faulty memory. When making changes to daily activities, be sure to do it gradually. Too many abrupt changes can be disorienting to an individual with AD or other forms of dementia, cause more stress, and lead to a hastening of the decline rather than slowing it.

As discussed in Chapter 6, games that use, and therefore strengthen, cognitive skills may be able to slow the progression of AD. Some great games for this purpose include crossword puzzles, word find games, Scrabble and other word games, trivia games, strategy games, cards, and video and computer games (Mayne, 2013).

Establishing Routine and Familiarity

Try to establish a regular routine, with meals, sleep, outings, and baths happening at about the same time each day. Schedule all doctors' appointments at roughly the same time if possible, such as first thing in the morning or early afternoon. It's important to organize the person's day around his or her sleep-wake cycle.

A person with AD will function more independently when the caregiver organizes the daily routine. Structured and pleasant activities can reduce agitation, improve mood, and decrease problematic behaviors. Planning activities for a person with dementia may require caregivers to make strides to organize the day, then explore, experiment, and adjust the schedule as necessary. To make a plan, attempt to determine the following (Alzheimer's Association, 2014d):

- The individual's likes, dislikes, strengths, abilities, and interests
- How the person normally structures his or her day
- What times of day the person has the least amount of problems and functions best
- The appropriate amount of time for meals, bathing, and dressing
- The best regular times for waking up and going to bed

It's also important to allow for flexibility within the daily routine for spontaneous activities.

As the disease progresses, the abilities of an individual with AD change and usually decline. This will require the caregiver to be creative and flexible and develop problem-solving strategies in order to adapt the daily routine to support these changes.

When creating a daily routine, develop a plan, write it down, and follow it. Alter the plan if it does not work and adjust to fit the needs of both the person with AD as well as the caregiver. In doing so, consider the following (Alzheimer's Association, 2014d):

- What activities work best? Which ones don't work well? Why? (Keep in mind that the success of an activity can vary from day to day.)
- Are there times when the person is encountering too much or too little stimulation (i.e., too much going on or too little to do)?
- Are spontaneous activities enjoyable and easily completed?
- Adjust the routine as the individual's abilities change.

Allow for periods of rest or just some down time. Don't be concerned about filling every minute with an activity.

The person with AD may need to balance activity and rest periods and may need more frequent breaks and varied tasks. If the individual appears bored, distracted, or irritable, it may be time to introduce another activity or to take time out for rest. The type of activity and whether a task is completed are not as important as the joy and sense of accomplishment the person gets from doing it. In the following tables are some suggested activities to consider when formulating a plan and an example of a daily plan.

Checklist of Daily Activities to Consider
• Household chores. Allow the person some responsibilities, but nothing too complicated and nothing that will compromise his or her safety. Responsibility will make the person more independent and decrease depression and problematic behaviors. • Meal times. • Personal care (e.g., bathing, brushing teeth, shaving, grooming, changing clothes). • Creative activities (e.g., music, art, crafts). • Intellectual activities (e.g., reading, puzzles). • Physical activity (e.g., exercise, toileting). If the person is incontinent, consider a timed toileting schedule every 2 to 3 hours during the day. • Social activity (e.g., having coffee with others, watching the news to learn about what is happening in the outside world). • Spiritual activity (e.g., prayers, quiet time for thinking).
From Alzheimer's Association, 2014d.

Daily Plan Example (For Early to Middle Stages of Alzheimer's)
Morning • Morning grooming: Wash face, brush teeth, get dressed • Prepare for breakfast: Set table and prepare food on plates, eat breakfast, clean up kitchen • Have coffee, make conversation

Daily Plan Example (For Early to Middle Stages of Alzheimer's) (continued)
Morning (continued)   • Do morning exercises   • Discuss the newspaper, try a craft project   • Take a break, have some quiet time   • Do some chores together   • Take a walk, play an active game
Afternoon   • Prepare for lunch: Set table and prepare food on plates, eat lunch, clean up kitchen   • Do non-demanding activity, such as listening to the news or to music, do crossword puzzles   • Do some straightening of the room, a little gardening, take a walk, visit a friend   • Take a short break or nap
Evening   • Prepare for dinner: Set table and prepare food on plates, eat dinner, clean up kitchen   • Talk or reminisce over coffee and dessert   • Do a non-demanding activity, such as play cards, watch a movie, give a massage   • Take a bath, get ready for bed, read newspaper or book
From Alzheimer's Association, 2014d.

Remember that the stimulation of new and different ideas and activities may refresh a person with AD and have positive effects, but too much change in the routine can be confusing and disorienting. Familiarity is very important to someone with AD or other forms of dementia. The stress of having to cope with sudden or significant change can make symptoms worse.

Safety

Safety should be a top priority in the household of an individual with AD. To maximize safety, the home should be surveyed, and some modifications may be necessary; however, the environment should remain familiar and uncluttered. Make sure to have ample lighting and clutter-free walkways, and keep harmful objects out of reach from the confused individual with AD (this includes cleaning solutions, bleach, medications, sharp knives, etc.). Other considerations may include putting locks on cabinets and ovens and unplugging dangerous appliances. Wandering behavior can be diminished with the installation of simple child-proof door knob covers, more complex door locks, or even in-house alarms or bells. Identification bracelets or necklaces may help minimize the hazardous consequences if wandering off does occur and the individual becomes lost. Decisions about driving generally rest on the judgment of family members, but in general, individuals with AD will eventually need to cease driving motor vehicles. Health care practitioners are encouraged consult local laws regarding their duty to report individuals who have conditions that may impair driving ability (Yaari & Corey-Bloom, 2007). See **Table 3-6** for some safety tips.

Environment

When a person has AD or another form of dementia, routine and a controlled environment are key to making his or her world as stress free as possible. As has been described earlier in this book, familiarity should be maintained in the environment of an individual with AD as much as possible. Try not to rearrange furniture or make drastic changes, so the person can feel more relaxed in familiar surroundings. Keeping the environment simple, uncluttered, and easy to maneuver through with as few changes as possible has been shown to diminish behavioral problems in individuals with dementia. See **Table 3-6** for details about how to create a safe and effective environment for someone with AD.

Staying Active

There are a variety of activities appropriate for people at every stage of dementia to assist in slowing the disease. Keep in mind that simply doing an activity is more important than the end result, even if the person had been a perfectionist or very goal directed before the onset of disease. Performing an activity has its own rewards and benefits. Following are some guidelines to keep in mind when selecting activities for someone with AD.

Guidelines for Therapeutic Activities
• Choose individualized activities that draw on past interests and skills • Choose activities that remind the person of his or her former occupation • Choose activities that stimulate the five senses: sight, hearing, taste, touch, smell • Choose activities that emphasize existing physical skills • Initiate the activity (and help the person along if necessary) • Ensure the person is willing to participate (ensure participation is voluntary) • Select intergenerational activities • Choose activities that appeal to both the facilitator and the person with dementia • Keep activities short

Activities should support a person's sense of self and bring out his or her skills, memories, and habits. They should also reinforce the person's sense of being in a group, which can provide friendship, mutual support, and connectedness with surroundings. There are a number of activities that may be beneficial, depending on the person and his or her level of functioning. Different activities may affect certain symptoms but not others; for example, dance therapy does improve balance and may improve appetite in some people but not others. It is preferable to plan activities the person would have

135

enjoyed when he or she was younger, to play on the person's remote memory. For example, consider any former hobby or interest, such as gardening, cooking, painting, drawing, singing, playing musical instruments, or listening to music.

Several programs that combine various therapeutic activities have shown favorable results in people with dementia. These include a multifaceted program of music, exercise, crafts, relaxation, dance, and structured sessions combining meditation, relaxation, sensory awareness, and guided imagery, "mind-over-body" techniques designed to calm and soothe (Rolland et al., 2008).

Many of the activities described in the following sections can be found in *The Alzheimer's Activities Guide: A Caregiver's Guide to Daily Activities for People with Alzheimer's Disease (In It Together)* (2005).

Outings

It is important for people with AD and other forms of dementia to go places with others. This keeps them connected with the world around them and helps them feel like they are still a part of a community. Unfamiliar places can be confusing and upsetting to individuals with dementia. It is important to structure any outing so the person is not overwhelmed and the outing is enjoyable.

The following are some examples of outings to consider. (Consider bringing a wheelchair on any outing if the person gets too tired from walking.)

- **Sporting events:** If professional games are too expensive, consider amateur games, such as minor league baseball or high school or college sports. There may be less pressure in buying the ticket, finding parking, and dealing with crowds. If the person is not having a good day, it will be less frustrating to change plans. If a live event is too stressful for the individual, consider watching a sporting event on television or listening to a radio broadcast.

- **Zoos:** Seeing exotic animals can be enjoyable. Consider asking the individual if he or she would like to see any particular animal. Limit excursions to one or two of the less crowded sections of the zoo, and consider the petting zoo as long as it is not too busy. Touching and having real interactions with animals can make the person feel connected with society and help with reminiscing about pleasant memories. Be aware of the animal's reaction to the person so he or she does not become frightened. If a trip to the zoo is too stressful, bring an animal to visit the person, such as a friendly and calm cat or dog. If the person is not apprehensive and reacts favorably, allow him or her to pet the animal. Also, walking a pet is good exercise and can be more pleasant than walking alone for individuals with dementia.

- **Art museums:** Visits to art museums can be visually stimulating and relaxing. Some museums have interactive exhibits that would allow the person to touch art. Walk through the exhibits and ask the individual about his or her thoughts and feelings about the artwork. Discuss colors and any associations the visit triggers. If a visit to an art museum is too stressful, consider excursions to a library and look at art books, or bring art books to the person. You could also set up pictures in a room of the house and stage an exhibit.

- **Fruit picking:** When choosing a location for picking fruit, choose one that is not too physically demanding or dangerous. Avoid fruit trees that require a ladder to get to the fruit or plants that have sharp thorns, such as blackberries or raspberries. Consider strawberry or blueberry farms or an orchard with smaller trees. Consider going to a fruit stand and allowing the person to help pick out the fruits and vegetables to bring home, and then wash them together. Enlist the person's ideas for making fruit pies or fruit salad.

- **Bowling:** Bowling stimulates hand-eye coordination and can be fun and foster team spirit. It may help with balance problems also. Help lift the ball and allow the person to assist with guiding it down the alley. Make sure the game is not competitive. Ask the bowling alley to put up bumpers for the gutter, and use the lightest ball. If bowling is too stressful, the person may wish to go to the bowling alley and watch and have discussions about the game.

- **Kite flying:** An inexpensive kite or one you make can be visually stimulating and allow the person to enjoy the outdoors. Be mindful of safety: Watch the weather, be careful about power lines, never use a metallic kite, and be aware of potential falling or tripping hazards. Consider getting the kite in the air and then allowing the person to hold the string. If flying a kite is too stressful, bring a comfortable chair for the person to sit in and watch the kite flying.

- **Boat watching:** Going to a harbor or lake to watch boats can be a very relaxing activity. Be mindful of safety around the water.

- **Libraries:** Looking at, reading, or simply touching books can be stimulating. Reading a book together or listening to a book on CD or tape is also enjoyable. Some libraries offer special events for elders. If the person has difficulty reading and comprehending, books with large pictures may be an alternative. Find a quiet, comfortable area to avoid distractions. Ask the person questions about the story or pictures while reading.

- **Visiting family and friends:** A short visit to see family members or friends can be a pleasurable activity that allows the person to interact with others and get out of the house. Being in familiar places may help trigger memories and stimulate conversations. If going to others' homes is too stressful, riding in the car around the block or having family and friends come visit the person may be enjoyable. Make sure visitors are aware of the individual's limitations, and have visitors come in groups of one to three, direct conversations to include the person, and do not carry on multiple conversations in the same room as the person.

Crafts and Hobbies

Helping create something can be extremely satisfying. This type of activity can foster hand-eye coordination and help maintain a person's motor skills. It can also tap into the individual's creativity. When individuals with AD can work with others, including those who also have AD or other forms of dementia, on art projects, this creates a partnership and fosters social interaction. The amount of interaction possible depends on how well both individuals can function. Following are some specific ideas.

- **Visiting a craft show:** Craft shows are great for interacting with others, stimulating all of the senses, and allowing someone with dementia to explore. Once at the show, allow the person to wander from table to table (with supervision) and discuss the things he or she sees. If going to a show would be too stressful or difficult, bring home craft magazines, how-to books, or things a person would see at a craft show and have one at home.

- **Pressing flowers and leaves:** This is a creative activity that combines physical activity, contact with nature, and visual skills. Gather leaves and flowers from a nature walk, making sure they are dry and avoiding moldy or rotten ones. If you don't press picked flowers right away, you may need to refrigerate them prior to use. Press them between two sheets of newspaper with heavy books on top, and allow leaves to flatten for 24 hours and flowers for about three days. If you wish, press a flattened flower or leaf between two sheets of wax paper with a warm iron for 10 seconds: Take care that the person with AD does not burn him- or herself.

- **Making a mobile:** Gather several lightweight objects of similar shape and size (such as shells, buttons, beads), lightweight string, and a plastic hanger. Tie the string around each object, leaving 6 inches of string on top, and allow the person to tie the objects to the hanger. The person can continue to add objects until he or she decides the mobile is complete. If the activity is too stressful, make the mobile yourself and allow the person to choose the order and placement of the objects. Be mindful of safety if the individual has a tendency to place objects in his or her mouth.

- **Stringing beads for bracelets or necklaces:** Use sturdy string and large beads that are colorful and easy to handle, but be careful the person does not put the beads in his or her mouth. Use a tape measure to determine the size of the wrist or neck, and make the string 6 inches longer than the measurement. Cut the string, tie one bead on the string 3 inches from the end, and then allow the person to add beads. You may need to demonstrate how to perform the task. If the activity is too stressful, allow the person to choose the colors and order of the beads as you place them on the string.

- **Making a birdfeeder:** All you need to make a birdfeeder are sturdy string, a pinecone, peanut butter, and birdseed. Tie a string at the top of the pinecone, apply peanut butter to the pinecone, and allow the person to roll the peanut-butter pinecone in the birdseed. Place the pinecone where the person can watch the birds come feed if possible. If this activity is too stressful for the person, talk through the steps and ask the person where the birdfeeder should be placed, preferably where the person can watch the birds come to feed. Talk about what kind of birds will come.

- **Creating a collage:** Gather safety scissors, photographs, sturdy board or corkboard, and a glue stick. Try to include pictures of family members, friends, or pets.

As you put the collage together, discuss who the people in the pictures are. If the individual is having difficulties recalling who they are, provide hints to trigger remote memories. If this activity is too stressful, allow the person to direct which pictures are used and where to place them as you create the collage and talk about who is in the photos.

- **Arranging flowers:** All that is necessary for this activity are flowers and a vase: Scissors are optional (you may cut the ends of the stems prior to having the person with AD help). Allow the individual to pick which flowers to use and arrange them in the vase. If this is too stressful, allow him or her to choose the flowers while you place them in the vase and talk about the flowers. Put the flower arrangement where the person can see it after completion of the activity.

- **Decorating a picture frame:** A homemade picture frame is a creative and constructive activity. The frame can be used by the person or given as a gift. Obtain an inexpensive frame, and use craft glue to attach buttons, shells, paperclips, peas, or any small objects to the front of the frame, making sure the person does not place the objects in his or her mouth. If this is too stressful for the person, allow him or her to direct you on what is put on the frame and where to put it. The person can decide when the project is complete. After the frame is dry, place a photo of something or someone of significance for the person in it. Colorful pictures from a magazine can also be used.

- **Playing with modeling clay or Play-Doh:** Get non-toxic modeling clay, which comes in a variety of colors, for the person to use to create something. Allow him or her to decide what to make, but if the individual does not have any ideas, suggestions can include paperweights, cups, or coin bowls. Play-Doh is softer and may be easier to work with than other types of clay. If this is too stressful, allow the person to direct what is made, and place the object where he or she can see it.

- **Making holiday cards:** Encourage the person to design a card and write the words for it. Offer suggestions and talk the individual through the activity if necessary. While making the card, talk about past holidays and the people to whom the card will be going. If the person has difficulty writing, ask him or her what you should write or allow the person to choose from a few pre-selected ideas.

Music

Music can be enjoyable, stimulate memory, and enhance verbal and visual skills. It can contribute to resynchronization (the stimulation of the timing processes within the brain), which can assist in improving the timing of motor actions, including walking or swinging the arms. Following are some suggested ways to use music with a person with AD.

- **Singing songs:** Give song lyrics to the person and encourage him or her to sing along with music or with other people. It may be helpful to offer the individual one sheet of music at a time. If this is too stressful or the individual can no longer read, just play the music and sing for him or her.

- **Going to concerts:** Look for concerts or music events that are of interest to the person. Many are free, and school choirs and church groups often offer free concerts for elders. If the person is unable to attend a concert, find a CD or tape of music he or she would enjoy listening to.

- **Playing a musical instrument:** If a person played a musical instrument in the past, ask if he or she would like to play again. Ask the individual to play a simple song or whatever comes to mind. If possible, provide musical accompaniment either by singing along, playing along, or using recorded music. If this is too stressful for the person, play the instrument for the individual or listen together to recorded music of the instrument the person used to play.

- **Dance:** Find recorded music from the person's past and have a dance. This activity helps strengthen muscles and preserve balance. While dancing, discuss memories the person has of dancing or thoughts about the song or ask questions about the music (e.g., "Is that a trombone or a trumpet?"). If this is too stressful for the person, give him or her a scarf, tambourine, or shaker and allow him or her to wave the object in time to music. Alternatively, the person can watch others dance and talk about dance and what it means to him or her.

- **Watching a musical:** Watching a musical movie from the individual's past is a great activity. The person can sing along or just enjoy watching. If he or she wishes, talk about the plot, make comments about the characters or actors, or talk about the scenery.

- **Listening to music from the past:** Popular music from one's past is often associated with happy events and can bring back important memories for a person. Many radio stations specialize in a specific era or genre, or you can obtain recorded music.

Nature

Contact with nature provides benefits to those with dementia, including physical exercise, fresh air, and stimulation of all the senses. Here are some suggestions for incorporating nature-oriented activities.

- **Gardening:** Planting a garden, weeding, raking leaves, and watering plants are all non-demanding activities an individual with dementia can do that can be fun and productive. Talk about what the plants are, when they will bloom, the type of fruits you will harvest, or whether the person thinks the plants need watering. If the individual is unable to perform gardening tasks, discuss gardening and specific flowers or plants or look at pictures of flora.

- **Taking nature walks:** Accompany the person on a walk and discuss the environment, scenic views, animals, and plants or leaves. Make sure to plan ahead and take necessary items, such as water and snacks. Choose a route that does not exceed the person's abilities: Avoid very long, strenuous walks. Consider taking a wheelchair in case the person tires. If this activity is too stressful, consider taking the individual into the yard and talking about the trees, squirrels, or cars driving by. If possible, make the route circular so the person ends back at the starting point, because it is sometimes difficult to make a person with dementia turn around to head back home.

- **Feeding fish, ducks, or birds:** A simple pleasure can be feeding animals, such as fish, ducks, birds, or squirrels. Bring old bread and allow the person to toss small pieces to the wildlife. Allow the person to sit if possible to prevent him or her from getting tired. Talk about the animals/birds, the weather, and your surroundings.

- **Collecting shells:** If you live near a beach, collecting shells can allow a person to observe nature and get some exercise. Make sure the ocean does not frighten the individual and that he or she can physically walk on sand. Talk about the shells and any memories from the person's past. If this is too stressful for the individual, consider getting a bag of shells from a craft store, pouring them on a table, and asking the person which ones he or she would like to place in a bowl or would like to collect. Alternatively, sit together near the beach and watch the ocean, birds, and people.

- **Bird-watching:** Bird-watching can be visually stimulating and allow the person to get outdoors. This can be done on a short walk, with the person in a wheelchair, or from a window. Place a birdfeeder where you wish to bird-watch to draw in birds to observe. Talk about the types of birds you see or get a bird-watching guide to help the individual identify different species.

- **Watching fish in a tank or birds in a cage:** Watching beautiful, multicolored fish swim or birds singing in a cage can be very relaxing and reduce anxiety. Another option is to have books or pictures of animals to look at or discuss with the person. Alternatively, a trip to the pet store can be a stimulating activity.

Helping Around the House

Individuals with dementia can develop feelings of uselessness and unproductiveness, which can cause depression and diminish quality of life. Keeping a person active and feeling as if he or she can contribute to household chores will help prevent this problem and bring about satisfaction. Performing simple household chores can make a person with dementia feel more independent and better about him- or herself and improve his or her quality of life. Following are some specific ways a person with AD can be involved in helping out around the house.

- **Helping with laundry:** Do laundry at the same time every day or on the same days of the week to establish a routine. Allow the person to take laundry out of the dryer, separate and match socks, fold clothes and towels, or organize clothes. Talk about memories from his or her earlier life, such as who did the laundry or whether he or she used a clothesline.

- **Polishing silverware:** This activity exercises motor skills. You may want to remove knives and separate forks and spoons to make this task easier and safer. Use a soft polish, and monitor the person for putting it in his or her mouth. After the polish has dried, buff off the cream and remove tarnish. If polishing is too difficult, have the individual separate and sort the silverware.

- **Sorting buttons:** Sorting, cleaning, and organizing activities can help keep a person busy and bring back memories from his or her past. Ask the individual to sort through a collection of buttons by shape, color, or size.

Alternatively, he or she can sort nuts and bolts from a toolbox, photos, or children's toys. Monitor the person to make sure he or she does not put objects in his or her mouth. If sorting is too difficult, ask the individual to tear paper into 6-inch strips and put them in a bowl. Demonstrate how to perform this task and then allow the person to continue.

- **Washing the car:** Ask the person to help wash, polish, or dry a car if he or she is physically able. Care should be taken to avoid spills and falls; make sure the person is not afraid of the water or getting sprayed. Do not worry about making a mess — clean up later. If it is too difficult for the person to help wash the car, have him or her keep you company while you wash it. Talk to the individual during this activity.

- **Washing fruits and vegetables:** Ask the person to separate fruits or vegetables. Ask him or her to wash them in preparation for meals or snacks. Alternatively, allow the person to set the table before meals. If in a facility, some individuals with dementia can assist other residents to the dining area.

- **Stamping envelopes:** Ask the individual to place stamps on envelops that need mailing. If this is too difficult, obtain rubber stamps, an ink pad, and some envelopes and allow the person to stamp the backs of the envelopes or on a piece of paper.

- **Helping at mealtime:** Activities the person may be able to do include beating eggs, decorating a cake, filling sugar or creamer bowls, kneading bread, and setting the table. Remember to provide step-by-step instructions and decide if it is safe for the person to be around knives or other sharp objects, mixers, and stoves.

- **Making the bed:** A daily routine can include having the person make his or her bed. This fosters a feeling of familiarity and comfort in repetition. Changing the sheets may be challenging, but if possible, it could be part of a routine for the person. If this is too stressful, allow the individual to help make the bed or just observe and direct while you make the bed.

- **Caring for houseplants:** This can be a pleasurable and relaxing activity and help a person feel productive. With help, the individual can do many of the tasks related to plant care, including repotting, watering or misting, and removing dead leaves or flowers.

Using Verbal Skills

Conversations can be frustrating for individuals with dementia. Normal exchanges with others can be loaded with information the person can no longer remember or recall. Activities that stimulate verbal skills can help the person reconnect with others. Following are some specific suggestions.

- **Reading a story aloud:** Reading newspapers, magazines, poems, or old letters is a good exercise. Individuals with dementia enjoy this type of routine and find it comforting. Make sure to keep distractions to a minimum by turning down the radio or television or doing the activity in a quiet area. You can obtain large-print publications from libraries and newspaper publishers. If the person is unable to read, read to him or her and ask questions about what is being read.

- **Geography:** Use a map or globe to stimulate conversations about islands, countries, or cities. Discuss types of animals that reside there, weather conditions, what you would wear there, or whether the person has ever been to that location. If he or she is unable to participate in such discussions, point out different places and talk about them while the individual listens.

- **Dictating a letter:** Ask the person to write a letter that you dictate or ask him or her what he or she would like to say to a family member or friend and assist the person in writing it. If this is too difficult or if the individual is unable to write, have him or her dictate a letter you will write.

- **Talking about historic events:** Because long-term memory is often intact with dementia, the person may find it enjoyable to discuss events from the past. Magazines that focus on history, such as *American Heritage* or *National Geographic*, or old books that have information and pictures may spur discussions and memories. You might also watch old videos of important moments or periods of history together. Remember that many old television series are now on DVD and can tap into a person's memories.

- **Asking for advice:** Elders usually love to give advice. This activity engages the person and allows him or her to contribute. Ask the individual's opinion or advice about a task, a person, a meal, or an activity. The question really does not matter — what matters is that you listen to the answer and show you are listening by asking questions and/or repeating what you think the individual said.

Games

Playing games can bring people together and reinforce social skills and good behavior. Individuals with dementia may not always remember the rules and may need to be prompted when it is their turn. Remember to be flexible with the rules if the person does not remember or becomes upset when corrected and reminded of the rules. The point of the game is the process of playing, engaging the person, and having fun. Following are some games to consider. Also see Chapter 6 for "brain games" to stimulate cognitive activity.

- **Bingo:** Use Bingo cards with large print, and when the number is called, say it verbally as well as showing a large picture of the number so the person can see it and hear it. You might consider playing in teams or having someone assist the person in playing. Provide small prizes, such as a photograph or tissues.

- **Crossword puzzles:** The caregiver could start a large-print crossword puzzle and ask the person for help.

Either have the person say the answers or fill them in him- or herself. If the person is unable to help provide answers or write, discuss the questions and think through the answers together.

- **Jigsaw puzzles:** Some jigsaw puzzles have large pieces and bright colors. Choose one with few pieces and simple designs. Ask the person to assemble the puzzle or hold a piece and ask him or her where he or she thinks it should go.

- **Word games:** Play find-a-word puzzles together or play the game yourself and point out the words you find to the person. Match U.S. presidents' first names with last names.

- **Tossing a ball or beanbag:** Find a comfortable place where the person can toss a ball or beanbag into a basket or through a large hole. You can modify this activity by throwing the ball or beanbag back and forth to each other, bouncing the ball back and forth, or having the person squeeze a stress ball.

- **Treasure hunt:** Fill a box with beans, corn, or rice and hide "treasures" in the box, such as buttons, coins, or any small objects. Be cautious the person does not place the objects in his or her mouth.

- **Draw a word:** Match a word with a picture: Either have the person do this or have him or her direct you as you work together.

- **Card games:** lay simple card games, such as Go Fish or Old Maid. Use large-print cards if possible. You can play a game where the person throwing down the highest card wins each hand. Very simple rules are best, but remember that a person with dementia may not always play by the rules, so be flexible and let him or her win. Sorting through postcards is also a good activity to stimulate memories.

Reminiscing

Remembering the past can be comforting and enjoyable for a person with dementia. Celebrating occasions is also a good way to trigger pleasurable memories and create new ones. Here are some ideas.

- **Celebrating a birthday:** Birthday celebrations bring people together and encourage reminiscing. The person can assist in preparing for the party and wish another person a happy birthday or just be the one who is celebrated.

- **Taking a picture together:** Bring out funny hats, colorful outfits, or pets with whom to have pictures taken. Take turns photographing each other and then enjoy the pictures together. Go to a photo studio to have pictures made, and then talk about the pictures (e.g., "Remember the day when we had this picture taken?").

- **Celebrating a holiday:** Go beyond celebrating the big holidays and celebrate the smaller ones (e.g., Arbor Day, Columbus Day, Mardi Gras, May Day, Flag Day), as well as special days you create. For Mardi Gras, have a parade and throw beaded necklaces and eat King Cake. For Arbor Day, plant or water a tree. For Columbus Day, read about Columbus. For May Day, make a May Day basket.

- **Putting a photo album together:** Bring out old photos and get pictures from magazines and newspaper articles and ask the person to help organize them into a collection and/or album. Create a story about each photo and write it down on a postcard or on the back of the picture for remembering later. Allow the person to organize the pictures in any fashion he or she wishes. Bring out the album later to allow the individual to reminisce. If he or she is unable to assist in this activity, have family or friends help you put one together, including stories about which you can talk to the person, and use the album periodically to remind the person of his or her life.

- **Stimulating memories about the person's past career:** Create a designated "office space" for the person to "work." He or she may be able to mimic some of the old tasks he or she used to perform and feel productive again. For example, if the person was an accountant, provide a desk and calculator; if he or she was a beautician, provide combs, brushes, and curlers. Make sure to supervise the work activities and ask for productivity reports or schedules, but when the person loses interest, remove the items and bring them out again at another time.

- **Fashion:** Talk about the type of clothes the person used to wear, ask about favorite outfits or colors, point out fashion in catalogues and magazines, and have the person assist in choosing outfits he or she will wear. Offer two to three choices to prevent overwhelming the person in making a decision.

- **Talking about childhood:** Reminiscing about childhood is often a very enjoyable activity for elders. Ask about where the individual was born, where he or she grew up and went to school, and how many brothers or sisters he or she had. Ask about favorite childhood memories or something that made the person laugh when he or she was a child. Be prepared for the individual to ask about relatives and friends who are no longer alive. Do not stimulate grieving by discussing their deaths unless the person wants to talk about this subject. If it seems to upset the person, allow him or her to discuss his or her feelings and/or distract his or her attention to another subject.

- **Watching old movies or television shows:** Watching old movies or TV shows can be fun and relaxing, as it allows a person to connect with old memories, reminds him or her of familiar stories, and is visually stimulating. You can find classic movies or TV series on public television, the Internet, Netflix, or cable channels, or on DVD. Choose movies or shows with which the person can connect.

Discuss the actors, the plot, or anything in the show that might be stimulating.

Pet Therapy

Pet therapy includes animal-assisted therapy and other activities involving animals. Animal-assisted therapy is a growing field that uses pets, including dogs, cats, birds, and fish, to help people better cope with physical and mental illness, including AD. Animal-related activities have the general purpose of providing comfort and enjoyment (Mayo Clinic, 2012b).

Imagine you're in the hospital and someone brings a dog to visit as part of a pet therapy program. You visit with the dog and its handler for 10 or 15 minutes, and you pet the dog and ask the handler questions. After the visit, you realize your mood is better and you're smiling. This makes you feel a little less tired and a bit more optimistic. Most people who participate in pet therapy can't wait to tell their family all about the experience and that charming animal. In fact, most begin looking forward to the pet's next visit (Mayo Clinic, 2012b).

The biggest concerns with pet therapy are safety and sanitation. Most facilities that use pet therapy have stringent rules to ensure that the animals are clean, vaccinated, well trained, and screened for problem behavior. Animal allergy is another consideration (Mayo Clinic, 2012b).

CHAPTER 8

FAMILY MATTERS

WHEN A PERSON DEVELOPS AD, MANY CHANGES OCCUR WITHIN THE FAMILY. THE PERSON WITH THE DISEASE AND THE FAMILY AS A WHOLE MUST DEVELOP AN UNDERSTANDING OF WHAT IS OCCURRING AND CREATE STRATEGIES TO MANAGE THESE CHANGES. CONFLICT CAN OCCUR WHEN FAMILY MEMBERS DO NOT WISH TO ACCEPT THE FACTS ABOUT THE LIKELY PROGRESSION OF DECLINE. THIS CHAPTER PRESENTS A DISCUSSION OF COMMON FAMILY ISSUES AND OFFERS SUGGESTIONS FOR THEIR MANAGEMENT.

Every individual with AD is a person, a member of a family, and plays a certain role in that family. And, every member of the family will be affected by the disease in some way. When a person is diagnosed with AD, the effects on that person and his or her family can be overwhelming. The reality that a spouse, a parent, someone you love has a devastating illness that could progress to the point at which he or she is no longer the person you once knew may cause conflict in the family and trigger a variety of emotions, including withdrawal, ignoring the problem, fear, sadness, confusion, and anger — maybe even rage. Conflicts are common as family members struggle to deal with the situation (Health Central, 2014).

Spouses, children, or other family caregivers may be reluctant to acknowledge the problem and seek help until a crisis arises that forces the family to seek outside assistance. Research has shown that it can take some families up to two years before asking for help to cope (Health Central, 2014). Initially, there seems to be a strong desire to live as if the problem did not exist and go on as if everything is the same. Roles change for caregivers as they begin taking on certain duties when the person with AD can no longer function independently. This usually occurs when at least one daily task needs to be done for the person, such as reminding him or her to take a shower or change clothes. Many family members need to assume more responsibilities they had not done previously; for example, a wife may have to start balancing the checkbook, a duty that was previously the husband's responsibility, or a husband may need to start doing laundry and cooking. The early stage of caregiving is marked by many struggles with admitting to and identifying the problems, altering day-to-day life to accommodate the individual's declining abilities, and negotiating decision-making, which may not be a smooth process for some caregivers.

Issues Caregivers May Deal With in Caring for Someone With Dementia
• Wants all my time and attention
• Makes constant unreasonable demands
• Is inflexible, critical, or negative
• Is unable to manage bills and finances but refuses to allow anyone to assist
• Refuses to take medications
• Complains about real or imagined physical symptoms
• Acts normal and charming in front of others but inappropriate at home
• Exhibits bizarre or inappropriate behaviors
• Has become suspicious or paranoid
• Experiences increasing memory loss
• Exaggerates or "cries wolf"
• Prefers to stay in bed and is "waiting to die"
• Refuses to allow others to assist with care
• Becomes furious when something does not go as he or she wishes
• Gets mad when told "no"
• Wants to eat constantly, not eat at all, or eat only one thing
• Refuses to take showers or change soiled clothing

Many family members reported experiencing frustration, resentment, grief, and loss of intimacy while at the same time experiencing increasing protectiveness and tenderness toward the person for whom they are caring. Spouses may begin to mourn the loss of their partner, including loss of intimacy, as roles shifted from a marital role to becoming a caregiver (Health Central, 2014). Children may feel resentment for the parent for consuming so much of their time or their inability to take on a traditional grandparent role.

Family Issues That Can Occur
• One spouse may refuse to share information about his or her spouse's physical health and mental abilities
• A family may refuse to accept the diagnosis of a dementing illness
• A sister may arrive from out of town and wish to dictate the way care for a parent is provided
• A son who visits once every 3 years may accuse the nursing home staff of neglect and mistreatment
• Relatives may argue during a time of crisis

Family members experience many different reactions as they interact with the individual with AD and with other caregivers and family members. Emotional maturity and intelligence are factors that affect how people will manage with the disease. Difficult decisions must be made and can profoundly affect the person with dementia as well as the family. In the face of these stressful situations, caregivers may become aware of strong and possibly conflicting feelings or may begin to change in their own behavior, role, and need to alter their activities and routine. Alternatively, caregivers may lack awareness of their own feelings and act out strongly. Feelings of anxiety, frustration, depression, and loss of control are common: They are normal and natural responses to these types of difficult situations.

Depression

Depression is a common occurrence among family members caring for an individual with AD or other forms of dementia. Sometimes, caregivers become sad and feel sorry for themselves, while at other moments, they are sad for the person with the disease. Caregivers may be fatigued and experience a lack of the energy that is needed to carry on a normal life, stay socially active, carry out daily activities, or pursue other activities that were once meaningful. In response to the new emotional and physical demands of providing care, caregivers may notice changes in their appetite or sleep habits and worry about the future.

Anger

Anger may emerge periodically. Family members may be angry and act out then feel badly for getting mad at someone they love who is sick. Frustration and anger are common occurrences and fairly normal feelings. The person with dementia may exhibit irritating behavior, seem ungrateful for the care that is provided, or be difficult to manage due to the cognitive decline. He or she may also act impulsively due to lack of control. Family members, particularly spouses, may be lonely and feel they have been deserted at a time in life when companionship seems very important.

Guilt

In response to conflicting feelings and a lack of ability to control the situation, guilt may develop. Guilt may be molded by previous beliefs, values, and experiences. Family members may wonder if they are doing enough or making the right decisions. Guilt may also arise over misunderstandings among family members.

Change and Uncertainty

Families should realize that change will occur and recognize that close relationships within the family that endure over time will have many nuances. Stress and uncertainty can be created when an illness touches a family, and each member of the family is affected differently. New emotions usually occur, and these changes are normal. Reaching out for help may assist families to cope and remain intact.

Role Changes
Adjusting to New Roles

Every person plays a role in the family, the community, and society. These roles are what define us as individuals and are the basis for all human relationships and interactions. Many people grow comfortable in their roles and come to depend on others to fulfill the roles that they play. In a family, people learn to rely on one another for certain things: A family may look to the grandmother to organize and prepare for holiday gatherings; a man may count on his wife to manage finances and pay bills; or a grown son may still turn to his aging parents for advice and emotional support. However, when an individual who previously played key roles in the family has dementia, the family dynamics will change. Intellectual, behavioral, or emotional changes that accompany a diagnosis of dementia can alter each person's ability to function in his or her predesigned roles. Families must be aware that these changes may occur and make adjustments accordingly.

Feelings of Loss

Feelings of loss are common for the person with AD and family members who are experiencing role changes. For individuals who have been accustomed to being in control, making decisions, and managing personal and financial affairs, the realization that they no longer are capable of doing these things and someone else is making decisions and performing certain

157

tasks may be upsetting. For family members and caregivers who must learn to assume different responsibilities, there may be anxiety, anger, or sadness about the situation. Sometimes cognitive impairment causes problems with an individual's ability to work, resulting in an unplanned early retirement and financial strain. A person with a diagnosis of dementia and his or her relatives may experience many adjustments and changes and a mixture of emotions. Families must cope with many losses and should work to create effective strategies that attempt to keep life as normal as possible while compensating for these losses of abilities, independence, function, and thinking, as well as the eventual loss of the person.

Intimacy: Sexual Functioning

Along with roles, sexual relationships may also change. The individual with dementia may no longer desire sexual contact, whereas a healthy spouse may still have needs and must struggle with feelings of rejection, anger, and frustration. Some people with AD experience an increased sexual desire and make excessive demands for frequent sexual encounters. The healthy spouse may no longer feel sexually attracted to the individual with dementia and may experience feelings of guilt. The caregiving role becomes more one of a friend or a parent than a partner and can result in a change in the nature of intimacy. Emotional bonding may undergo changes as the person's behavior changes. Caregivers may also feel that the individual with dementia is selfish and unappreciative, which can further cause issues with emotion, sexuality, and roles.

Difficulties in Social Situations
Embarrassment

Some families may attempt to protect the person who has AD in social situations. A family member may try to compensate or "cover up" for the person's forgetfulness, changing behaviors, or diminished social skills. Filling in missing words and diverting the focus of attention away are common maneuvers of caregivers. Experiencing a sense of discomfort or embarrassment is normal, and deciding what to tell friends and acquaintances may be difficult.

Isolation

Other dilemmas that families face include whether the individual with dementia should be isolated to avoid difficult situations. Should the person with AD and his or her family continue normally as if nothing had changed? There are no easy answers. Some situations may be more stressful than others. The goal is to keep the affected individual as socially active as possible, with attention paid to the physical and psychological safety of the family, especially children. Social isolation of a person with dementia may lead to a lower level of functioning or increased confusion.

Social Effects on the Healthy Spouse

Spouses of individuals with AD must face some alterations in their social lives. Healthy spouses may realize that some friends and acquaintances will visit less often, it is harder to enjoy going out, or the affected spouse may be less affectionate. When someone has dementia, changing his or her routine or frequently traveling to new places can be disruptive, and this may impact the social life of the person as well as the spouse. Each spouse must develop a comfortable strategy suitable to meet his or her own needs for social involvement, as well as the continuing needs of the affected partner. Just because the individual with dementia can't continue certain social activities, his or her spouse does not have to stop — changes can be made to meet the emotional and social needs of both partners; for example, someone else could stay with the individual with dementia to allow the spouse time away to socialize. Every person requires time for him- or herself, time for work, and time for leisure. Breaks or periods of time away from the individual with AD can re-energize caregivers, allowing them to continue caring for the person.

Sharing the Burden

Social altercations are one of the most difficult aspects of the dementia for family members. Lost social skills may cause the individual with AD to act impulsively and lash out, which can make loved ones feel hurt and sad. Those who are closest may experience a strong mix of feelings as changes occur and the person behaves differently. This is understandable, because people grow to love one another based largely on social traits, such as sense of humor, kindness, and special interests. Talking with family or friends, support groups, or professionals may help family members cope. Families and friends may draw together to provide mutual support or can become divided, depending on the situation and each individual's stage of understanding and acceptance. Many experience a grieving process over the loss of the person they once knew even before physical death occurs. Getting support and being able to vent frustration and sadness can ease the burden. When the responsibility of care is shared, tasks may be more bearable.

To Tell or Not to Tell

Sometimes families choose not to tell others because they are embarrassed by AD or by the affected person's behaviors or symptoms. They hide problems with memory, cognition, and other areas by becoming more isolated and avoiding social engagements. Another issue to consider is the belief that friends and family would label the individual with dementia or treat him or her as "less than" equal. What's more, some families believe that others would not be able to accept the situation and would "fall apart" if they knew, so they keep the disease a secret to spare others the burden of knowing.

Trying to keep AD a secret requires a great deal of effort and may result in stress to the affected individual and/ or caregiver. Others who interact with the person with AD are aware that he or she is having problems but are unsure of how to respond. Discussing the situation openly often reduces stress and anxiety for all parties involved, including the person with dementia, family, and friends.

If one wants to enlist the aid of friends and neighbors, they can be more helpful once they have a clear understanding of the problem. In new social situations, everyone may feel more relaxed if they are prepared before interacting with the affected person and understand what his or her difficulties are and how they can make the situation most comfortable.

Talking to Children About Dementia

Young children may need to know that the person with dementia may exhibit behavior that is not a reflection of anything they have done. If children understand that a grandparent is sick, they are less likely to believe that he or she does not remember their names because he or she does not love them.

How to Tell

An issue with which families are confronted is how to explain to others that their loved one has dementia. A young child may not understand why his grandparent behaves rudely and curses. Friends may be confused about why the person and his wife no longer go to social gatherings. Some friends and family members have trouble accepting the individual as "sick," since the person may appear physically healthy. There are no "right" or "wrong" ways to tell others about the illness — the best way will vary from one situation to the next and from one family to another. Some families feel it is important to emphasize that the individual has a neurological illness and not a mental illness or emotional disorder. In general, the best method is to be truthful and give a simple explanation (Northwestern University, 2012).

Thinking About the Future

As the person with dementia's abilities decline and he or she becomes more disabled, independent living, even with the help

161

of a caregiver, becomes more difficult. Making the decision that more care is needed and considering a move to a different setting, such as a nursing home, requires time and considerable planning. This may ultimately be a reasonable solution to caring for an individual with AD in order to meet his or her physical and emotional needs.

When is it time to consider a nursing home for someone with dementia? Many families agonize over this decision. Husbands, wives, or adult children who have worked to keep the individual with dementia at home may feel obligated to continue providing in-home care and may feel a sense of failure and guilt when they begin to consider nursing home placement. Each situation is different, and the person's health status and each family member's ability to maintain the person at home will vary due to many factors, such as his or her level of functioning, the availability of community resources, and the health and energy level of family members to provide care. Because of all these considerations, no fixed guidelines can dictate when nursing home care should occur.

Safety is the most important factor to consider when making decisions regarding care. When staying at home without supervision is dangerous, alternatives should be considered. If a person lives alone and begins to forget to turn off the gas or wanders off, his or her safety may be in danger. The health of the caregiver must also be considered, because caregiving causes stress (emotional as well as physical), which may cause declines in the caregiver's health (Northwestern University, 2012).

Although whether to consider out-of-home care is a very important decision, it's not the only one families must make. Following are additional decisions that must be made.

Decisions to Be Made in Caring for Elders with Dementia
Relocation: When will it be necessary, and where to relocate? • Relative's home • Assisted living facility • Nursing home
Driving: When to limit or stop driving? How to accomplish this? Who will be the driver and caregiver for the person who is no longer driving?
Financial and legal issues: What are the costs of care and living arrangements? What resources are available to pay for care? Who will make decisions regarding care of the person with dementia?
Daily care: Who will assist with daily care, including bathing, grooming, eating, toileting, and other household activities? Who will manage finances and daily expenses? Who will make the decisions regarding health care?
End-of-life care: Who will make decisions regarding continuity of care and end of life?

In most families, there is generally one individual who will assume the role of primary caregiver and decision maker, but there are always others involved in making decisions. Conflicts and disagreements can occur when emotions are involved. Other issues to consider include lack of understanding regarding AD, an inability to accept the deterioration of an individual's abilities and cognitive status, and dysfunctional family relationships. The process of making decisions about care is discussed in more depth in Chapter 9.

Family Conflict

Family members may disagree about care choices for their loved one with dementia. There may be arguments among family members, they may ignore the problems that are obvious, they may blame others for their loved one's behaviors or decline, or they may attempt to change many of the decisions that have already been made. Any or all of these behaviors can occur and can lead to conflict between family members or between families and health care providers.

To manage conflict within a family, certain steps can be taken to find a solution. Begin by figuring out what the problem is: a lack of knowledge regarding the disease or the individual's declining abilities? Role conflict among family members? Inability to afford care for the person with AD? It may help to ask the questions listed in the following table. The key to resolving family conflict is to define the problem and learn its meaning as identified by the family members involved. It may also help to investigate previous methods that family members have used to resolve conflict. Next, identify and organize resources that may be available within the family and from outside resources. Additional suggestions are listed in the second table.

Questions to Ask When Difficult Decisions Must Be Made
What is the problem? Whose problem is it? Who's to decide? What's to be done? Who's to do it? When should it be done? Where should it be done? How should it be done?

Ways to Manage Family Conflict
Communication Crisis intervention Problem solving Education Social support Conflict resolution Family therapy

Additional Suggestions for Families in Managing Care
Sharing Responsibility

Ideally, family members should share the responsibility in care. In some cases, this does not occur. Caregivers should consider each family member's preferences, resources, and abilities, including physical, mental, and financial. Some family members may be able to provide hands-on care, either in their own homes or in the individual's home. Others may be more comfortable with respite care, household chores, or errands. Still others may be better suited for handling financial or legal issues (Alzheimer's Association, 2014f).

Regular Meetings

Talking or meeting regularly can assist families in caring for someone with AD. If there are issues a family is unable to discuss, family conflict is present, or additional resources are necessary, counselors or other family conflict management sources may need to be involved. Optimally, plan regular face-to-face family meetings or phone conferences to discuss the person with dementia and any issues that are affecting him or her and the family. It is advisable to include everyone who is part of the family and the caregiving team, including family friends and other close contacts. Discuss each person's caregiving responsibilities and challenges and decide whether and how to make changes accordingly. If time, distance, or other logistical problems are issues for certain family members, consider sharing through email updates with the entire family or start a family blog (Alzheimer's Association, 2014f).

Honesty and Respect

Be honest and talk about feelings in an open, constructive manner to help defuse tension. If certain family members are feeling stressed or overwhelmed, they should be encouraged to let others know, and then the family should work together to brainstorm and find more effective ways to share the burden of care. All involved should be careful to express feelings without blaming or shaming anyone else. Avoid using "I" statements, such as, "I'm having trouble juggling my own schedule with all of Dad's appointments." Families should keep an open mind when listening to other family members share their thoughts and feelings.

Don't criticize — there are many "right" ways to provide care. Respect the abilities, style, and values of each family member and caregiver. Be especially supportive of family members who are responsible for daily, hands-on care, because this can be a difficult and sometimes thankless job.

Counseling

Consider counseling if the stress of caring for someone with AD is too much and is tearing the family apart. Remind family members to seek help when the pressures of the disease, care, and life in general become too great. Families should be encouraged to consider joining a support group for Alzheimer's caregivers or seeking family counseling. Remember, working through conflicts together can help move families on to more important things like caring for the person with dementia and enjoying their time together as much as possible.

CHAPTER 9

TAKING CARE OF BUSINESS

THIS CHAPTER ELABORATES ON WAYS TO MANAGE LEGAL AND FINANCIAL AFFAIRS, AS WELL AS HOW A PERSON MAY PLAN FOR HIS OR HER HEALTH CARE THROUGH ADVANCE DIRECTIVES.

"Taking care of business" when one has AD involves making good decisions about one's health, health care and legal and financial affairs. Some of these decisions can be made by the person with AD when he or she is in the early stages of disease, and other decisions will be made by caregivers and others.

Physical Health

Living a healthy life and staying independent are important goals for most individuals. However, when someone develops AD, staying independent may remain a priority initially, but the ability to be independent and make important decisions may need to change as the situation changes and the individual's abilities decline. The priority of living a healthy life may change to living well and focusing one's energies on what is most important. Educating oneself on AD and ways to slow its progression and taking a proactive approach to living are the best strategies for living well. Focus on maintaining physical, emotional, social, and spiritual health. Learn to anticipate and understand the expected changes that will occur, acknowledge and accept the changes, and learn to adjust and cope with them. Adopt a healthy lifestyle by eating well, exercising, and getting regular checkups from a health care practitioner who is knowledgeable and trustworthy.

Creating a Care Team

It is important to create a care team of family, friends, neighbors, professionals, and community support services. Identify a trusted decision-maker. Often this person is a family member or friend. The individual with AD should have a conversation with this person about the type of help that may be needed and what the long-term priorities are to be. The care team should include the following:

- The person with AD
- Family members, whether living with the affected person or elsewhere
- Close friend(s)
- Neighbors or others who may help with day-to-day tasks
- A general practitioner, neurologist, counselor, and/or other specialist experienced in care of people with AD
- Volunteers from community organizations and members of a church or other social group

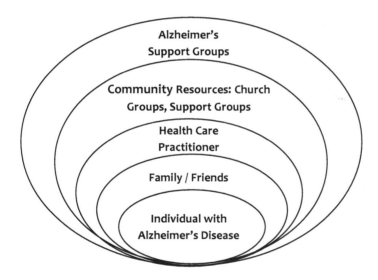

The person who has AD is the center of the care team and will always be the primary concern of the team. Tips to remember when developing the care team include the following:

- Identify which friends, family, and neighbors are capable and willing to help.

- When asking for help, seek individuals who are willing to listen and who care.
  Avoid people who seem judgmental, critical, or blaming.
- Discuss the situation and the help that will be needed: Have a conversation with each person of the care team to explain the expectations of his or her role, the expected changes in the individual with AD, and the affected person's wishes for the direction of care and his or her life.
- Be specific in expectations of what help is needed or may be needed in the future from each care team member. This should be stated plainly.
- Family and friends should be asked to do normal activities with the affected individual, such as shopping or preparing meals.
- If someone isn't able to help, don't blame him or her. He or she may not be capable of providing the help needed or may have other things going on in his or her life.
- Be appreciative and say thank you! Everyone likes to feel appreciated, and thanking people makes it more likely that they will help again in the future.

Organizing Important Documents and Information

It is normal for someone with a diagnosis of AD and his or her family to feel overwhelmed, but even so, it is important to take care of business by paying attention to the details of legal matters and planning for health care needs. The person should take time to review important information, put together a comprehensive business plan, and have conversations with care partners and/or family members about the legal plans that are being put into place.

As soon as possible after an individual is diagnosed with AD or another dementia, he or she should make a list of the important documents that will need to be in place. Reviewing the list with family members will allow the person to be involved in making decisions about these documents and help the caregiver and family members to be aware of his or her wishes. These documents should include the following:

- Personal paperwork, such as birth certificate and marriage or divorce papers
- Banking, investment, and retirement information (e.g., name of bank manager and financial consultant, bank account locations and numbers, checkbooks, monthly bank statements and investment statements, pension plans, retirement savings plans, user names and passwords for any online banking or investment accounts)
- Lawyer's name and contact information
- Information about previous employers
- Health records
  » Medicare and/or Medicaid card
  » Doctors' names and contact information
  » List of current medicines, allergies, medical history, past surgeries
  » Medicare supplement insurance information
  » Medicare part D medicine plan
- Mortgage information (e.g., lender name and contact information)
- Insurance policies (e.g., whether death and/or disability insurance is in place, other types of policies [e.g., homeowners, car, life, long-term care, burial] and policy issuers, beneficiaries)
- Home/car ownership (e.g., bill of sale, titles, duplicate titles, notice of transfer and release of liability, smog certification)
- Prepaid funeral arrangements and/or cemetery plot
- A will that states how property should be divided after the person's death

- A document that names a substitute decision-maker who can make decisions about financial and legal matters on the person's behalf when he or she is no longer able to

- A document that names a substitute decision-maker for future health care decisions

- A "living will" or advance directive that describes the person's wishes for health care and end-of-life care in the future to help the family make difficult decisions that may arise during the course of the disease when the person is no longer able to make these decisions for him- or herself

Contact a lawyer for information about state-specific requirements regarding legal documents, or contact the closest Alzheimer's Association chapter.

Paying For Care

Paying for medical and long-term care services can be a major issue for families. Resources for paying for care may include Medicare, Medicaid, Social Security Disability, programs for veterans with AD, private health insurance, long-term care insurance, and savings/out of pocket. Understanding what is covered by Medicare or other sources and what an individual may have to pay out of pocket will help families prepare for the often significant cost that can accompany caregiving (Alzheimers.gov, n.d.).

People who are younger than 65 years and have AD can apply for Social Security Disability. The Social Security Administration recently added Early-Onset Alzheimer's Disease as one of the conditions that qualifies for the Compassionate Allowance Program. This program helps speed the processing of applications of people with certain conditions. Information on how to apply for Social Security and the Compassionate Allowance Program is available online.

Competency and Consent

Making valid health care decisions requires a person to have a certain level of cognitive capacity. *Capacity* usually means

171

that the individual is rational and able to make decisions based on his or her own wishes and values. Capacity in the case of AD means that the person must understand the important risks and benefits of the proposed choice or plan of care and other options available and must be able to make decisions and communicate what his or her choices would be. A person who can do these things can make a valid decision regarding approval or rejection of his or her health care treatment (Berg, 2013).

In individuals with AD, competency will change over time: There will be an overall decline, but capacity will also fluctuate from one day to the next. The key to assessing capacity to make decisions and choices depends on several factors:

- The type of decision being made and the degree of importance of the decision
  » Life-threatening/life-saving decision, such as placing a feeding tube or taking a medication at that moment
  » Preference, such as whether to take a bath today or not
- The level of orientation and understanding a person demonstrates at that moment

Health care practitioners are obligated by law and medical ethics to get the informed consent of their patients before initiating any type of care or treatment. Pertinent information must be given to a competent individual who is capable of making a voluntary choice. However, when a person with AD lacks the competence to make a valid decision about treatment, an alternate person may be chosen to make decisions for him or her. Because the degree of competency and ability to make decisions of someone with AD will vary day to day, it can be difficult in some cases to determine if the person is legally able to give consent. When possible, it is preferable to allow the individual to look far into the future and make as many decisions in his or her own care as possible (Berg, 2013).

Advance Planning

One way a person can make decisions about the direction of his or her health care while he or she is still able to make rational decisions is through advance directives (sometimes referred to as *living wills*). This allows a person to make decisions ahead of time, knowing that a point will come at which he or she will no longer be able to make rational decisions. Creating an advance directive encompasses taking an in-depth look into the health care decisions that may be presented as a person's abilities decline and his or her care needs become more complex.

Some individuals who chose not to pursue advance directives and are no longer able to make rational decisions will need another individual to make decisions regarding health care choices, referred to as the surrogate decision-maker, or health care proxy. The surrogate decision-maker is selected to make health care decisions and is legally assigned this right through a written authorization to represent or act on another's behalf in private affairs, business, and legal matters. A court determines who the health care "power of attorney" agent will be when the person with AD does not wish a family member to make his or her health care decisions and/or is no longer capable of making rational choices. If a person is unable to make rational choices and resists having a power of attorney assigned, then two health care practitioners must determine the individual to be incompetent and a court must agree in order to have a power of attorney assigned against the person's wishes.

Note that a person assigned power of attorney is able to make both legal decisions and health care decisions unless the courts determine that different individuals will perform these functions. In some cases, one person makes legal decisions (e.g., manages assets, finances) and another makes health care decisions.

Making plans for the future is guided by three principles: autonomy, beneficence, and non-maleficence. The most important principle in determining the direction of one's life is autonomy (or self-rule). It means that, while the person is able to make rationale choices, he or she should make decisions regarding his or her own life and thus determine what type of care to pursue (or not pursue) and his or her own destiny. This self-determination should be respected as much as possible and for as long as possible while the individual is able to make rational choices. Consideration must be given not only to deciding how a person will live his or her own life but also to balancing the need to promote good for the person and prevent harm. Often, the person and his or her care team are making these decisions together. Initially, the direction of care will be looked at globally:

- What type of disease prevention strategies will be pursued?
- What type of diet, exercise, and lifestyle factors will be considered?
  - » Brain-stimulating activities
  - » Vitamins, alternative therapies
  - » Health care visits to maintain health
- What type of disease slowing strategies will be pursued?
  - » Diet, exercise, lifestyle
  - » AD screening (early detection)
  - » Medications to slow the disease progression (e.g., acetylcholine inhibitors, NMDA, antidepressants) and medications for managing behavioral issues
- How will issues be managed as the disease progresses?
  - » Stopping an individual from driving a motor vehicle
  - » Managing depression if necessary
  - » Managing behavioral problems if necessary
  - » Managing other health issues (e.g., unstable gait/falls, dysphagia, weight loss)
- How aggressive will care be? What type of care? How will end-of-life issues be handled?
  - » Nursing home or assisted living facility placement
  - » Hospitalizations
  - » Feeding tube placement, if necessary

» Aggressive types of care when infections occur, including aggressively managing respiratory infections
» Intubation/mechanical ventilation, if necessary
» Feeding tube placement for inability to maintain weight, dysphagia, weight loss

As previously mentioned, the level of competency of an individual with AD, and thus his or her ability to make decisions, will vary from day to day and moment to moment. Decisions regarding health care can be weighed on a significance scale that takes into account the type and seriousness of each decision (i.e., life-threatening or just preference), the affected person's level of competency at that moment in time, and his or her past and present wishes regarding health care, as spelled out in an advance directive. As much as possible, the person's mental well-being should be maintained through small-scale moment-to-moment interactions and experiences that enhance and encourage as much independence as possible.

Important Decisions to Be Made

A variety of issues in the life of an individual with AD must be considered when making preparations for future care; these issues are best considered earlier rather than later. It may be hard to consider some of these issues and questions at first, because this means thinking about a time when the individual is well advanced into the disease. However, looking ahead, making decisions, and putting preparations in place early may help allow for a smoother transition for everyone. Depending on the person's level of cognition and stage of disease when he or she is diagnosed with AD, allow him or her as much autonomy and participation in decision making as possible for as long as possible. If the person's dementia is at a more advanced stage, those involved with making decisions should at least try to act on what the person's wishes would be. Note that much of the information in this "Important Decisions" section was taken from a website on dementia and Alzheimer's care by Russell and colleagues (2013).

Who Will Make Decisions?

Questions to consider in preparing for Alzheimer's and dementia care include deciding who will make health care and/ or financial decisions when the person is no longer able to do so and what the person's wishes are. It is a good idea to write them down on paper so they will be preserved and respected by all members of the family.

Care team members should consider meeting with an attorney to understand the best options available. They should also consider designating and filing legal paperwork for power of attorney, for both financial matters and health care. If the person has already lost competency and the capacity to make rational decisions, caregivers should apply for guardianship/ conservatorship.

How Will Care Needs Be Met?

Team members must decide how care needs will be met. Sometimes family members assume that a spouse or nearest family member can take on caregiving, but that may not always be the case. Caregiving is a big commitment that becomes more demanding over time. The person with AD may eventually need around-the-clock care. Family members must consider their own health issues, jobs, and responsibilities to others. Communication is essential to make sure that the needs of the person are met and that the caregiver has the necessary support to meet those needs.

Where Will the Person Live?

It is also important to decide where the person will live. Is his or her own home appropriate, or is it difficult to access or make safe for later? If the person is currently living alone, for example, or far from any family or other support, it may be necessary to relocate him or her or consider a facility with more support. Care team members will need to find out what options for care are available. In some areas, a person can hire a care manager privately. Geriatric care managers can provide an initial assessment and assistance with managing a person's case, including crisis management, interviewing in-home help, and placement in an assisted living facility or nursing home.

Developing a Daily Routine

As was discussed earlier in this book, having a general daily routine for a person with AD or other forms of dementia helps caregiving run smoothly. The routine does not have to be rigid or set in stone, but will give a sense of consistency, which is beneficial to the person even if he or she can't communicate it. Familiarity can help give the person with AD some degree of stability and control in his or her life. Every family will have their own unique routines, especially regarding daily tasks, socialization, contact with family and friends, and ways of communication. Still, it is important to attempt to maintain the person's past daily routine as much as possible. Keep a sense of structure. Try to keep consistent daily times for activities such as waking up, meal times, bathing, dressing, receiving visitors, and bedtime. Keeping these activities at the same time and same place can help orient the person.

Let the person with AD know what to expect in a simple, straightforward manner and make sure that he or she understands. Consider establishing cues to signal the different times of day. For example, in the morning, open the curtains to let sunlight in. In the evening, put on quiet music to indicate it is bedtime.

Involve the person in daily activities as much as he or she is able to be involved. For example, a person may not be able to tie his or her shoes but may be able to put clothes in the hamper. Digging in the yard may not be safe, but the person may be able to weed, plant, or water. Judgment should be used in determining what is safe and what the person can handle. Note that much of the information in this section was taken from a website on dementia and Alzheimer's care by Russell and colleagues (2013).

Visitors and Social Events

Visitors can be a rich part of the day for an individual with AD. Having others visit can also provide an opportunity for the caregiver to socialize or take a break. Plan visits at a time of day when the person can best handle them. Visitors can be briefed on communication tips if they are unfamiliar with how to communicate with someone with AD or are uncertain about what to do or say. Visitors can bring memorabilia, such as a favorite old song or book.

Family and social events may be appropriate, as long as the person with Alzheimer's is comfortable. Focus on events that won't overwhelm the person; too much activity or stimulation at the wrong time of day might be too much to handle, leading to the occurrence of behavioral problems. Note that much of the information in this section was taken from a website on dementia and Alzheimer's care by Russell and colleagues (2013).

Handling Challenges in Caregiving

As has been discussed throughout this book, one of the most painful aspects of AD is watching a person with the disease display behavior he or she never would have previously or that even seemed possible. AD can cause substantial changes in how an individual acts. This can range from the embarrassing, such as inappropriate outbursts, to hallucinations, paranoia, and violent behavior. In making decisions about AD care, caregivers should become increasingly vigilant for the person's safety in the home as he or she loses his or her memory and experiences declines in cognitive and physical abilities. Everyday tasks like eating, bathing, and dressing can become major challenges. As challenging behavior progresses, caregivers may find themselves too embarrassed to go out or to seek help. Unfortunately, difficult behavior is often part of AD. Part of "taking care of business" may involve team members seeking help from medical practitioners and reaching out to caregiver groups for support. Note that much of the information in this section was taken from a website on dementia and Alzheimer's care by Russell and colleagues (2013).

Considering Long-Term Care

AD is a progressive disease that worsens over time as memory deteriorates. In the advanced stages, around-the-clock care is often necessary. Thinking ahead to this possibility can help make decisions easier. Every family is different, but knowing the options available can help a family make an informed decision. Options for long-term care include hiring in-home help, day programs, respite care, and nursing homes. Note that much of the information in this section, "Considering Long-Term Care," was taken from a website on dementia and Alzheimer's care by Russell and colleagues (2013).

Options for Care at Home

In-home help refers to professional caregivers who are hired to provide assistance for an individual with AD in his or her place or residence. In-home help ranges from assistance for a few hours a week to live-in help, depending on the individual's needs. Evaluate what sort of tasks are needed, how much the individual can afford to spend, and what hours are needed. Getting help with basic tasks like housekeeping, shopping, and other errands can help provide more focused care for the person.

Another option when a person with AD lives at home is participation in *day programs*, also called *adult day care*. These programs typically operate on weekdays and offer a variety of services, from activities and socialization opportunities to medical care and physical therapy. They also provide a chance for caregivers to continue working or attend to other needs. When considering programs, it may be best to focus on those that specialize in dementia care.

An additional option when a person with AD lives at home is *respite care* — short-term residential care. The person with AD stays in a facility temporarily, which gives the caregiver a block of time to rest, travel, or attend to other things.

Considering a Change in Living Arrangements

The physical and mental demands for care will increase as AD progresses, the individual's abilities decline and health care needs increase. The demands on the caregiver may become overwhelming — it may get to the point where physical tasks like bathing, dressing, and toileting may require total assistance by the caregiver. The level of supervision required also increases with time, and it may get to the point when the caregiver may not be able to leave the individual with AD alone. Nighttime behaviors may disrupt the person's sleep, making it difficult for the caregiver to sleep. With some individuals, belligerent or aggressive behaviors may be more than a caregiver is able to manage, or the caregiver may not feel safe (Russell et al., 2013).

For these reasons, it may be necessary to consider moving the person to a facility, such as a nursing home or assisted care facility. If the health and safety of either the caregiver or the person with AD is being compromised, an alternative living arrangement and/or care options may be best. If the person with Alzheimer's is living alone or the primary caregiver has health problems, moving the person to a facility may need to be considered sooner rather than later. It is important to consider whether health and safety can be balanced with other obligations, either financial or to other family members; for example, will an individual with AD be able to afford appropriate in-home coverage if a family member or friend cannot continue caregiving? The care team should investigate options and determine when a change or move is necessary (Russell et al., 2013).

When the decision to move the person has been made, the first step is finding the right place. An important consideration is location: A location that is convenient to the family will make it easier for family members to visit and have more opportunity to be involved in care and monitor the care being provided. However, sometimes due to availability or financial reasons, it is not possible to find a facility that is close (Alzheimer's Association, 2014c).

It is important to visit all facilities under consideration to make an informed choice. Care team members should be comfortable with the care the facility provides and be able to form relationships with the staff so that everyone can work together to provide the best care (Alzheimer's Association, 2014c). First impressions will probably be the look and feel of the facility. The following are important issues to investigate:

1. Is the facility clean, well kept, and odor free?

2. Are the rooms spacious enough, attractive, and pleasant?

3. Is the furniture comfortable and in good repair?

Once the physical characteristics of a nursing home have been assessed, the care team should try to determine the level of care provided. Look for signs of how personable the staff members are and whether they show respect, dignity, and compassion. Are the residents of the nursing home up, dressed, and well groomed, or are they physically restrained and overmedicated?

Some nursing homes are designated for the care of people with dementia or have units to meet the special needs of those with dementia or other cognitive impairment. If a caregiver is trying to get an individual with AD admitted to a particular facility, the initial visits will probably be spent with the admissions or marketing person and include a tour of the facility. Once it is determined the location is right and there are available beds, it may be helpful to go by the facility unannounced to get a feel for how it runs. It will also be helpful to speak with the coordinator of the AD program (if the facility has one) and spend time in the actual unit where the people with AD live. Staff members who work with people with Alzheimer's should be asked the following questions about the program and services (Alzheimer's Association, 2014c):

- What kinds of activities are provided for people with memory loss? How many hours a day do the residents have planned activities? How many days a week does the facility provide activities? (The better programs have structured activities throughout the day, at least five days a week.)

- What makes the dementia unit specialized?

- What precautions are provided for those who wander? What safeguards does the facility provide, and is it possible for someone to walk out?

- Does the staff have special training for dealing with difficult behaviors?

When a caregiver is choosing a facility, he or she may consider speaking with the family members of other residents who are in that facility. It may also be helpful to look closely at the residents to see if any of them are similar to the person with regard to stage of disease, personality and other factors to try to determine how well he or she may fit in (Alzheimer's Association, 2014c).

Some facilities do not have dedicated staff for individuals with AD. This does not necessarily mean that the facility should not be considered, since the facility may still be able to meet the needs of the individual and family in other ways. However, even when a facility does not have staff dedicated to people with AD, it is important to speak with the staff members who actually work with the residents, such as the Activities Coordinator or the Recreation Director. It may be helpful to ask what activities the facility offers and how individuals with AD can and do participate (Alzheimer's Association, 2014c).

Other considerations for deciding on a facility that will provide long-term care include the following (Alzheimer's Association, 2014c):

1. As the disease progresses and the individual with AD declines, will the facility be able to accommodate his or her needs?

2. Will this setting still work in six months or a year, or will a change be necessary? Does the facility have a relationship with other facilities that provide care for people in the

later stages of the disease? If so what are the names of those facilities?

3. It is very important to review admission and discharge criteria. Under what conditions might a resident be asked to move (e.g., change in behavior, change in financial circumstances)? Even though most placements work out, be aware that some do not.

REFERENCES

Aboukhatwa, M., Dosanjh, L., & Luo, Y. (2010). Antidepressants are a rational complementary therapy for the treatment of Alzheimer's disease. *Molecular Neurodegeneration, 5* (10), 1–17.

Aliev, G., Obrenovich, M., Reddy, V., Shenk, J., Moreira, P., Nunomura, A., Zhu, X., Smith, M., & Perry, G. (2008). Antioxidant therapy in Alzheimer's disease: Theory and practice. *Mini Reviews of Medicinal Chemistry,* 8(13), 1395–1406.

Alzheimer Society of Canada. (2012). Impact of the disease. Retrieved February 2, 2014 from http://www.alzheimer.ca/en/About-dementia/Alzheimer-s-disease/Impact-of-the-disease

The Alzheimer's Activities Guide: A Caregiver's Guide to Daily Activities for People With Alzheimer's Disease (In It Together). (2005). Forest Pharmaceuticals, Inc., St. Louis, MO & Cincinnati, OH.

Alzheimer's Association. (2014a). Alternative treatments. Retrieved February 2, 2014 from https://www.alz.org/alzheimers_disease_alternative_treatments.asp

Alzheimer's Association. (2014b). Alzheimer's facts and figures. Retrieved February 2, 2014 from http://www.alz.org/alzheimers_disease_facts_and_figures.asp

Alzheimer's Association (2014c). Choosing a care facility. Retrieved February 2, 2014 from http://www.alz.org/nyc/in_my_community_17490.asp

Alzheimer's Association. (2014d). Creating a daily plan. Retrieved January 27, 2014 from http://www.alz.org/care/dementia-creating-a-plan.asp

Alzheimer's Association. (2014e). Mild cognitive impairment. Retrieved February 2, 2014 from http://www.alz.org/dementia/mild-cognitive-impairment-mci.asp

Alzheimer's Association. (2014f). Resolving family conflict. Retrieved February 2, 2014 from http://www.alz.org/care/alzheimers-dementia-family-conflicts.asp

Alzheimer's Association. (2014g). Stay socially active. Retrieved March 9, 2014 from https://www.alz.org/we_can_help_remain_socially_active.asp

Alzheimer's Association (2014h). Treatment horizon. Retrieved February 2, 2014 from http://www.alz.org/research/science/alzheimers_treatment_horizon.asp

Alzheimer's Association (2014i). What is Alzheimer's? Retrieved February 2, 2014 from http://www.alz.org/alzheimers_disease_what_is_alzheimers.asp

Alzheimer's Association (2014j). Younger/early onset Alzheimer's & dementia. Retrieved February 2, 2014 from http://www.alz.org/alzheimers_disease_early_onset.asp

Alzheimers.gov. (n.d.). Paying for medical care and daily living services. Retrieved February 1, 2014 from http://www.alzheimers.gov/paying.html

Anderson, H. S. (2014). Alzheimer disease. Retrieved February 2, 2014 from http://emedicine.medscape.com/article/1134817-overview

185

REFERENCES

Annweiler, C., Llewellyn, D., & Beauchet, O. (2013). Low serum vitamin D concentrations in Alzheimer's disease: A systematic review and meta-analysis. *Journal of Alzheimer's Disease*, 33(3), 659–674. doi: 10.3233/JAD-2012-121432.

Bennett, D., Schneider, J., Buchman, A., Barnes, L., Boyle, P., & Wilson, R. (2012). Overview and findings from the Rush Memory and Aging Project. *Current Alzheimer Research*, 9(6), 646–663.

Berg, S. (2013). Consent & competency with Alzheimer's. Retrieved February 1, 2014 from *http://www.ehow.com/about_6390092_consent-competency-alzheimer_s.html*

Bianchetti, A., Rozzini, R., & Trabucchi, M. (2003). Effects of acetyl-L-carnitine in Alzheimer's disease patients unresponsive to acetylcholinesterase inhibitors. *Current Medical Research Opinions*, 19(4), 350–353.

Bird, T. D. (2012). Early-onset familial Alzheimer disease. In Pagon, R. A., Adam, M. P., Bird, T. D., et al., (Eds.), GeneReviews™ [Internet]. Seattle: University of Washington. Retrieved February 2, 2014 from *http://www.ncbi.nlm.nih.gov/books/NBK1236/*

Braunstein, G. D. (2012). Alzheimer's disease and dementia: For seniors, a prevention puzzle tougher than any Sunday crossword but clues, hope abound. *The Huffington Post*, Retrieved February 2, 2014 from http://www.huffingtonpost.com/glenn-d-braunstein-md/alzheimers-prevention_b_1923481.html

Breslau, E. (n.d.). 7 foods that reduce your Alzheimer's risk. Retrieved February 2, 2014 from http://www.grandparents.com/health-and-wellbeing/health/foods-reduce-alzheimers-risk

Brewer, G. (2009). The risks of copper toxicity contributing to cognitive decline in the aging population and Alzheimer's disease. *Journal of the American College of Nutrition*, 28, 238–242.

Bright Focus Foundation. (2013). How the brain and nerve cells change during Alzheimer's disease. Retrieved February 2, 2014 from http://www.brightfocus.org/alzheimers/about/understanding/brain-nerve-cells.html

Brown, E., Raeu, P., Halpert, K., Adams, S, & Titler, M. (2009). Evidence-based guideline detection of depression in older adults with dementia. *Journal of Gerontological Nursing*, 35(2), 11–15.

Byrd, L. (2011). *Caregiver survival 101: Managing the problematic behaviors in individuals with dementia*. Eau Claire, WI: PESI Publishing.

Chapman, R., Mapstone, M, Porsteinsson, A., Gardner, M., McCrary, J., DeGrush, E., Reilly, L., Sandoval, T., & Guillily, M. (2010). Diagnosis of Alzheimer's disease using neuropsychological testing improved by multivariate analyses. *Journal of Clinical and Experimental Neuropsychology*, 32(8), 793–808.

Chen, K., Reese, E., Kim, H., Rapoport, S., & Rao, J. (2011). Disturbed neurotransmitter transporter expression in Alzheimer's disease brain. *Journal of Alzheimer's Disease*, 26(4), 755–766.

186

Chintamaneni, M., & Bhaskar, M. (2012). Biomarkers in Alzheimer's disease: A review. *ISRN Pharmacology*, 2012 June 28. Retrieved February 2, 2014 from http://www.ncbi.nlm.nih.gov/pmc/articles/PMC3395245/

Chow, T., Pollock, B., & Milgram, N. (2007). Potential cognitive enhancing and disease modification effects of SSRIs for Alzheimer's disease. *Neuropsychiatric Disease and Treatment*, 3(5), 627–635.

Craft, S. (2009). The role of metabolic disorders in Alzheimer disease and vascular dementia: two roads converged. *Archives of Neurology*, 66(3), 300–305.

de Jager, C. A., Oulhaj, A., Jacoby, R., Refsum, H., & Smith, A. (2012). Cognitive and clinical outcomes of lowering homocysteine-lowering B-vitamin treatment in mild cognitive impairment: A randomized controlled trial. *International Journal of Geriatric Psychiatry*, 27, 592–600.

DeNoon, D. J. (2005). Obesity and Alzheimer's: High insulin levels linked to Alzheimer's. Retrieved February 2, 2014 from http://www.webmd.com/alzheimers/guide/20050808/obesity-alzheimers-risk

Dezell, M., & Hill, C. (2013). The nervous system. Retrieved February 2, 2014 from http://www.netplaces.com/alzheimers/what-is-alzheimers-disease/the-nervous-system.htm

Douaud, G., Refsum, H., de Jager, C. A., Jacoby, R., Nichols, T. E., Smith, S. M., & Smith, A. D. (2013). Preventing Alzheimer's disease–related gray matter atrophy by B-vitamin treatment. *Proceedings of the National Academy of Sciences of the United States of America*, 110, 9523–9528.

Ellul, J., Archer, N., Poppe, M., Boothby, H., Nicholas, H., Brown, R., & Lovestone, S. (2007). The effects of commonly prescribed drugs in patients with Alzheimer's disease on the rate of deterioration. *Journal of Neurology, Neurosurgery, & Psychiatry*, 78(3), 233–239.

Engelhart, M. J., Geerlings, M. I., & Ruitenberg, A. (2002). Diet and risk of dementia: Does fat matter? The Rotterdam Study. *Neurology*, 59, 1915–1921.

Exigence Group. (2012). Poor sleep linked to Alzheimer's disease risk factors. Retrieved February 2, 2014 from http://www.theexigencegroup.com/news/intelligence/article:poor-sleep-linked-to-alzheimer-s-disease-risk-factors-/

Gestuvo, M., & Hung, W. (2012). Common dietary supplements for cognitive health. *Aging Health*. 8(1), 89-97.

Gilbert Guide (n.d.). Validation therapy, redirection: Creative techniques for talking to a loved one with dementia. Retrieved February 2, 2014 from http://www.psgdc.org/GG_article1.html

Greenstein, R. (n.d.) Mediterranean diet pyramid. Retrieved February 2, 2014 from http://oldwayspt.org/resources/heritage-pyramids/mediterranean-pyramid/overview

Gutierrez, D. (2013). B vitamins slow progression of Alzheimer's: Study. *Natural News*. Retrieved March 9, 2014 from http://www.naturalnews.com/040787_b_vitamins_alzheimers_dementia.html

Hachinski, V., Oveisgharan, S., Romney, A. K., Shankle, W. R. (2012). Optimizing the Hachinski Ischemic Scale. *Archives of Neurology*, 69(2), 169–175.

Health Central. (2014). Family caregivers often delay seeking assistance until crisis points. Retrieved February 2, 2014 from http://www.healthcentral.com/alzheimers/news-25914-5.html

Honea, R., Thomas, G., Harsha, A., Anderson, H., Donnelly, J., Brooks, W., & Burns, J. M. (2009). Cardiorespiratory fitness and preserved medial temporal lobe volume in Alzheimer disease. *Alzheimer Disease and Associated Disorders*, 23(3), 188–197.

Kapoor, M. C. (2011). Alzheimer's disease, anesthesia and the cholinergic system. *Journal of Anesthesiology Clinical Pharmacology*, 27(2), 155–158.

Kawahara, M., & Kato-Negishi, M. (2011). Link between aluminum and the pathogenesis of Alzheimer's disease: The integration of aluminum and amyloid cascade hypotheses. *International Journal of Alzheimer's Disease*, March 8. Retrieved February 2, 2014 from http://www.ncbi.nlm.nih.gov/pmc/articles/PMC3056430/

Kennard, C. (2006). Clock Drawing Test. Retrieved March 9, 2014 from http://alzheimers.about.com/od/diagnosisissues/a/clock_test.htm

Kluger, J. (2010). The impact of Alzheimer's disease by the (very scary) numbers. *Time*, Sept 23. Retrieved February 2, 2014 from http://healthland.time.com/2010/09/23/the-impact-of-alzheimers-disease-by-the-very-scary-numbers

Konkel, L. (2013). Can hormones stave off Alzheimer's disease? Retrieved February 2, 2014 from http://www.livescience.com/27123-hormone-therapy-alzheimer-risk.html

Laino, C. (2007). Estrogen therapy may protect the brain. Retrieved February 2, 2014 from http://www.webmd.com/alzheimers/news/20070502/estrogen-therapy-may-protect-brain

Laitinen, M. H., Ngandu, T., Rovio, S., Helkala, E. L., Uusitalo, U., Vitanen, M., et al. (2006). Fat intake at midlife and risk of dementia and Alzheimer's disease: A population-based study. *Dementia and Geriatric Cognitive Disorders*, 22(1), 99–107.

Luchsinger, J. A., Tang, M. X., Shea, S., & Mayeux, R. (2002). Caloric intake and the risk of Alzheimer's disease. *Archives of Neurology*, 59, 1258–1263.

Maki, P., Perschler, P., Dennerstein, L., Clark, M., Henderson, V., Guthrie, J., Vogrin, S., & Resnick, S. (2005). Hyperlipidemia as a risk factor for cognitive impairment: Evidence from fMRI studies in midlife women. *Alzheimer's & Dementia: The Journal of the Alzheimer's Association*, 1(1), S77–S78.

Masterman, D. (2003). Treatment of the neuropsychiatric symptoms of Alzheimer's disease. *JAMDA Supplement*. S146-S154.

Mayne, D. (2013). Brain games for Alzheimer's. Retrieved February 2, 2014 from http://www.livestrong.com/article/35946-brain-games-alzheimers

MayoClinic. (2014a). Can exercise prevent Alzheimer's disease? Retrieved March 9, 2014 from http://www.mayoclinic.org/diseases-conditions/alzheimers-disease/expert-answers/alzheimers-disease/faq-20057881

Mayo Clinic. (2013). Diabetes and Alzheimer's linked. Retrieved February 2, 2014 from http://www.mayoclinic.com/health/diabetes-and-alzheimers/AZ00050

Mayo Clinic. (2014b). Diagnosing Alzheimer's disease. Retrieved March 9, 2014 from http://www.mayoclinic.org/diseases-conditions/alzheimers-disease/basics/tests-diagnosis/con-20023871

Mayo Clinic. (2012a). Heart-healthy diet: 8 steps to prevent heart disease. Retrieved January 27, 2014 from http://www.mayoclinic.com/health/heart-healthy-diet/NU00196

Mayo Clinic. (2012b). Pet therapy: Man's best friend as healer. Retrieved January 27, 2014 from http://www.mayoclinic.org/pet-therapy/ART-20046342?pg1

Merck. (2013a). The Merck Manual Home Health Handbook: Dementia. Retrieved February 2, 2014 from http://www.merck.com/mmhe/sec06/ch083/ch083c.html

Merck. (2013b). The Merck Manual Home Health Handbook: Genes and chromosomes. Retrieved February 2, 2014 from http://www.merckmanuals.com/home/fundamentals/genetics/chromosomes_and_genes.html

Mini-Mental State Exam (MMSE) (n.d.). *Wikipedia*. Retrieved February 2, 2014 from http://en.wikipedia.org/wiki/Mini%E2%80%93mental_state_examination

MoreFocus. (n.d.). Alzheimers disease treatment hormone therapy. Retrieved February 2, 2014 from http://www.tree.com/health/alzheimers-disease-treatment-hormone-therapy.aspx

Morris, M. C., Evans, E. A., Bienias, J. L., Tangney, C. C., Bennett, D. A., Aggarwal, N., et al. (2003). Dietary fats and the risk of incident Alzheimer's disease. *Archives of Neurology, 60*(2), 194–200.

Morris, M. C, Evans, D. A., Tangney, C. C., Bienias, J. L., & Wilson, R. S. (2006) Associations of vegetable and fruit consumption with age-related cognitive change. *Neurology, 67*(8), 1370–1376.

Musicco, M., Palmer, K., Salamone,G., Lupo, F., Perri, R., Mosti, S., Spalletta, G., di Iulio, F., Pettenati, G., Cravello, L., & Caltagirone, C. (2009). Predictors of progression of cognitive decline in Alzheimer's disease: The role of vascular and sociodemographic factors. *Journal of Neurology, 256*(8), 1288–1295.

National Institute of Neurological Diseases and Stroke (2014). NINDS Alzheimer's Disease Information Page. Retrieved February 2, 2014 from http://www.ninds.nih.gov/disorders/alzheimersdisease/alzheimersdisease.htm

National Institute on Aging. (2004). Low free testosterone levels linked to Alzheimer's disease in older men. February 2, 2014 from http://www.nia.nih.gov/espanol/newsroom/2004/01/low-free-testosterone-levels-linked-alzheimers-disease-older-men

National Institute on Aging (2012). Alzheimer's disease fact sheet. Retrieved February 2, 2014 from http://www.nia.nih.gov/alzheimers/publication/alzheimers-disease-fact-sheet

National Institutes of Health (n.d.). Alzheimer's disease. Retrieved February 2, 2014 from http://www.nlm.nih.gov/medlineplus/alzheimersdisease.html

National Institutes of Health (2010). Neurons, brain chemistry, and neurotransmission. In *The brain: Understanding neurobiology*. Retrieved February 2, 2014 from http://science.education.nih.gov/supplements/nih2/addiction/guide/lesson2-1.htm

National Sleep Foundation. (2013). How much sleep do we really need? Retrieved February 2, 2014 from http://www.sleepfoundation.org/article/how-sleep-works/how-much-sleep-do-we-really-need

NCCAM-NIH. (2013). Dietary supplements and cognitive function, dementia and Alzheimer's disease: What the science says. Retrieved February 2, 2014 from http://nccam.nih.gov/health/providers/digest/alzheimers.htm

NCCAM-NIH. (2008). Grape seed extract may help prevent and treat Alzheimer's. Retrieved February 2, 2014 from http://nccam.nih.gov/research/results/spotlight/062408.htm

Northwestern University. (2012). The family's response. Retrieved February 1, 2014 from http://www.brain.northwestern.edu/patients/family.html

Paddock, C. (2013). Exercise may ward off Alzheimer's and Parkinson's. Retrieved February 2, 2014 from http://www.medicalnewstoday.com/articles/267396.php

Peterson, A. (2004). New treatments for Alzheimer's symptoms: To curb aggression, paranoia in dementia patients, doctors turn to schizophrenia drugs. *The Wall Street Journal*, August 26. Retrieved February 2, 2014 from http://www.globalaging.org/health/us/2004/alz.htm

Peterson, R. (2011) Mild cognitive impairment. *New England Journal of Medicine*, 364, 2227–2234.

Phillips, B. (2007). Alzheimer's disease: Can we slow the progression? Retrieved February 2, 2014 from http://ezinearticles.com/?Alzheimers-Disease---Can-We-Slow-the-Progression?&id=865807

Physician's Committee for Responsible Medicine (2013). Dietary guidelines for Alzheimer's prevention. Retrieved February 2, 2014 from http://www.pcrm.org/health/reports/dietary-guidelines-for-alzheimers-prevention

Radiological Society of North America. (2007). High blood pressure may heighten effects of Alzheimer's disease. Retrieved February 2, 2014 from http://www.sciencedaily.com/releases/2007/11/071128114847.htm

Ramachandran, T. (2013). Alzheimer's disease imaging. Retrieved February 2, 2014 from http://emedicine.medscape.com/article/336281-overview

Raschetti, R., Albanese, E., Vanacore, N., & Maggini, M. (2007). Cholinesterase inhibitors in mild cognitive impairment: A systematic review of randomised trials. *PLOS Medicine*, 4(11), e338. doi:10.1371/journal.pmed.0040338.

Rattue, P. (2011). Alzheimer's disease impact on caregivers: New study. Retrieved February 2, 2014 from http://www.medicalnewstoday.com/articles/236750.php

Rodrigue, K. M., Rieck, J. R., Kennedy, K. M., Devous, M. D. Sr, Diaz-Arrastia, R., & Park, D. C. (2013). Risk factors for β-amyloid deposition in healthy aging, vascular and genetic effects. *JAMA Neurology*, 70(5), 600–606.

Rolland, Y., Abellan van Kan, G., & Vellas, B. (2010). Healthy brain aging: Role of exercise and physical activity. *Clinical Geriatric Medicine*, 26(1), 75–87.

Rolland, Y., Abellan van Kan, G., & Vellas, B. (2008). Physical activity and Alzheimer's disease: From prevention to therapeutic perspectives. *Journal of the American Medical Directors Association*, 9(6), 390–405.

Rondeau, V., Jacqmin-Gadda, H., Commenges, D., Helmer, C., & Dartigues J-F. (2009). Aluminum and silica in drinking water and the risk of Alzheimer's disease or cognitive decline: Findings from 15-year follow up of the PAQUID cohort. *American Journal of Epidemiology*, 169, 489–496.

Rosack, J. (2002). SSRI improves behavior symptoms in demented elderly patients. *Psychiatric News*, 37(7), 28.

Russell, D., de Benedictis, T., & Saisan, J. (2013). Dementia and Alzheimer's care: Planning and preparing for the road ahead. Retrieved February 2, 2014 from http://www.helpguide.org/elder/alzheimers_disease_dementias_caring_caregivers.htm

Salzman, C., Schneider, L., & Alexopoulos, G. (2000). Pharmacological treatment of depression in late life. In Bloom, F. E. & Kupfer, D. J. (eds). *Psychopharmacology: The Fourth Generation of Progress*. New York: Raven Press. Retrieved March 9, 2014 from http://www.acnp.org/g4/GN401000141/CH.html

Sanders, L. (2011). Antidepressants show signs of countering Alzheimer's: Mice and human data link treatment to less plaque in the brain. *ScienceNews*, 180(6), 5.

Scarmeas, N., Luchsinger, J., Schupf, N., Brickman, A., Cosentino, S., Tang, X., & Stern, Y. (2009). Physical activity, diet, and risk of alzheimer disease. *Journal of the American Medical Association*, 302(6), 627–637.

Schwartz, J., Allison, M., Ancoli-Israel, S., Hovell, M., Patterson, R., Natarajan, L., Simon J. Marshall, S., & Grant, I. (2013). Sleep, type 2 diabetes, dyslipidemia, and hypertension in elderly Alzheimer's caregivers. *Archives of Gerontology and Geriatrics*, 57(1), 70–77.

Scott, P. S. (n.d.). Slowing Alzheimer's progress: How to slow the progression of Alzheimer's disease. Retrieved February 2, 2014 from http://www.caring.com/articles/slowing-alzheimers-progress

Smith, M., Wayne, M., & Segal, J. (2013). Alzheimer's & dementia prevention: How to reduce your risk and protect your brain. Retrieved February 2, 2014 from http://www.helpguide.org/elder/alzheimers_prevention_slowing_down_treatment.htm

Sofi, F., Macchi, C., Abbate, R., Gensini, G., & Casini, A. (2010). Effectiveness of the Mediterranean diet: Can it help delay or prevent Alzheimer's disease? *Journal of Alzheimers Disease*, 20(3), 795–801. doi: 10.3233/JAD-2010-1418.

Solomon, A., Kivipelto, M., Wolozin, B., Zhou, J., & Whitmer, R. (2009). Midlife serum cholesterol and increased risk of Alzheimer's and vascular dementia three decades later. *Dementia and Geriatric Cognitive Disorders*, 28, 75–80.

Stankiewicz, J., & Brass, S. (2009). Role of iron in neurotoxicity: A cause for concern in the elderly? *Current Opinion in Clinical Nutrition & Metabolic Care*, 12, 22–29.

Steenhuysen, J. (2012). Hormone replacement therapy may cut Alzheimer's risk in menopausal women. Retrieved February 2, 2014 from http://vitals.nbcnews. com/_news/2012/10/24/14678558-hormone-therapy-may-cut-alzheimers-risk-in-menopausal-women?lite

Thompson, S., Lanctot, K., & Herrmann, N. (2004). The benefits and risks associated with cholinesterase inhibitor therapy in Alzheimer's disease. *Expert Opinion on Drug Safety*, 3(5), 425–440.

University of Maryland Medical Center (2012). Alzheimer's disease. Retrieved February 2, 2014 from http://umm.edu/health/medical/reports/articles/alzheimers-disease

University of Texas at Dallas. (2013). Hypertension could bring increased risk for Alzheimer's disease. Retrieved February 2, 2014 from http://www.utdallas. edu/news/2013/3/19-22631_Hypertension-Could-Bring-Increased-Risk-for-Alzhei_article-wide.html

USCF Memory and Aging Center (n.d.). Mild cognitive impairment. Retrieved February 2, 2014 from http://memory.ucsf.edu/education/diseases/mci

Veracity, D. (2005). How acetyl-L-carnitine prevents Alzheimer's disease and dementia while boosting brain function. Retrieved February 2, 2014 from http://www.naturalnews.com/015553.html#ixzz2hqKNAQyM

Wadsworth, T., Bishop, J., Pappu, A., Woltjer, R., & Quinn, J. (2008). Evaluation of coenzyme Q as an antioxidant strategy for Alzheimer's disease. *Journal of Alzheimer's Disease*, 14(2), 225–234.

WebMD. (2014) DHEA Supplements don't help Alzheimer's: Hormone has no effect on Alzheimer's disease. Retrieved March 9, 2014 from http://www. webmd.com/alzheimers/news/20030407/dhea-supplements-dont-help-alzheimers

WebMD. (2014). Vinpocetene. Retrieved March 9, 2014 from http://www.webmd. com/vitamins-supplements/ingredientmono-175-VINPOCETINE.aspx?activeI ngredientId=175&activeIngredientName=VINPOCETINE

Weuve, J., McQueen, M. B., & Blacker, D. (2014). The AlzRisk database. *Alzheimer Research Forum*. Retrieved February 2, 2014 from http://www.alzrisk.org/

Whiteman, H. (2013). Lack of sleep may increase Alzheimer's risk. Retrieved February 2, 2014 from http://www.medicalnewstoday.com/articles/267710.php

Yaari, R., & Corey-Bloom, J. (2007). Alzheimer's disease. *Seminars in Neurology*, 27(1), 32–41. Retrieved February 2, 2014 from http://www.medscape.com/viewarticle/553256_8

ABOUT THE AUTHOR

LISA BYRD, PhD, FNP-BC, GNP-BC, Gerontologist

Lisa Byrd is a seasoned practitioner and gerontologist with a diverse nursing background that includes extensive work in geriatric advanced practice nursing. Dr. Byrd is currently Director of Clinical and Facility Compliance with Provider Health Services, LLC. In this capacity, she oversees physicians and nurse practitioners working at long term care and skilled nursing facilities in several states.

In addition to speaking nationally on a variety of health care topics, Dr. Byrd is an adjunct professor at the University of Mississippi Medical Center and the University of South Alabama, teaching courses in the graduate nursing programs. She is also a published author, a section editor for *Geriatric Nursing Journal*, and a successful business owner.

Dr. Byrd shares her expertise with the Alzheimer's Foundation of America as a member of the credentialing team for the "Excellence in Dementia Care Program," offering facility certification in dementia care.